PENTOXIFYLLINE

:

A VERSATILE OFF-PATENT MEDICINE
BEST NOT OVERLOOKED

:

OVERVIEW WITH EXTENSIVE BIBLIOGRAPHY

Robert Charles Powell, MD, PhD

North Charleston, SC:
CreateSpace Independent Publishing Platform, 2015
Copyright © 2015
Robert Charles Powell

ISBN-10: 1511673052
ISBN-13: 978-1511673051
First Edition: April 2015
10 9 8 7 6 5 4 3 2 1

PENTOXIFYLLINE:

A VERSATILE OFF-PATENT MEDICINE BEST NOT OVERLOOKED

> OVERVIEW

Key Words: inflammation, immune modulation, steroid sparing,
             TNF-alpha, PDE-4, IL-6, AChEI,
             brain, kidney, heart, liver, lung, cancer, infection

Abstract: While pentoxifylline [pen-tox-IF-i-lin] shares some properties with other xanthenes – especially its much more potent precursor "pentifylline," its R-1 metabolite "lisofylline," its more potent S-1 metabolite "hydroxypentoxifylline," and the deuterated S-1 metabolite analogue "CTP-499" – **pentoxifylline stands out for its balance of positive physiologic actions.** Since pentoxifylline ("Trental") went "off patent" in the United States in 1998, research on it has risen dramatically – for example, from 656 known medical articles in 1995 to 2,533 articles as of 2014. Efforts continue toward finding a better, safer – and patentable – nonselective phosphodiesterase (PDE) inhibitor, or selective PDE-4 inhibitor, or selective acetylcholinesterase inhibitor (AChEI), or tumor necrosis factor (TNF) alpha synthesis inhibitor (rather than "blocker"), or plasma interlukin-6 (IL-6) suppressor, or leukotriene synthesis inhibitor, or protein kinase A (PKA) activator, or macrophage-derived nitric oxide synthase blocker, or matrix metalloproteinase (MMP) 2 & 9 inhibitor, or chitinase inhibitor, or malondialdehyde antagonist, or adenosine A2a receptor agonist as the pivotal role of inflammation in disease gains new appreciation. **In case after case, pentoxifylline emerges perhaps not as the strongest but as the safest alternative with the fewest side-effects. Its role as an augmenter of less safe or more expensive medications also grows year by year.** The original characterization of pentoxifylline as a medication for treating "intermittent claudication" has become almost irrelevant — except in so far as that diagnosis is appreciated as indicating systemic inflammatory disease. **Pentoxifylline enhances both survivability and general well-being through multiple pathways.** [Extensive endnotes document the main text.]

Considering that pentoxifylline [pen-tox-IF-i-lin], a metabolite of the markedly more potent pentifylline [pen-tIF-i-lin], first arrived on the clinical scene over 40 years ago, in 1972 – and went off-patent in the United States well over a decade ago, in 1998 – it continues to generate a notable and increasing amount of research worldwide. Currently there is major interest in the cardiopulmonary, renal, and hepatic uses of pentoxifylline, but virtually every medical specialty has seen articles published on pentoxifylline in recent years if not recent months. Briefly stated, pentoxifylline appears to "enhance survivability" in a wide variety of clinical situations. It certainly ranks high on the list of medications to pack if one anticipates being stranded on a desert island – or in the midst of a war. Pentoxifylline indeed was on the list of essential emergency medications during the Cold War concern about radiation effects from nuclear bombs, the later concern about severe acute respiratory syndrome (SARS), the last decade of concern about avian influenza ("bird flu"), and the more recent concern about H1N1 influenza ("swine flu"). Late in 2005 the US government alone proposed to purchase eighteen and a half million tablets of time-release pentoxifylline for use by current and former service members, and, given the recent burst in clinical research interest, one has to imagine that the size of future purchases will increase; indeed, pentoxifylline was in short supply in the US during the first ten months of 2010. Think about that for a moment: why did US pharmacies start running out of pentoxifylline, forcing even the manufacturer of the more expensive brand-name version to ramp up production? Consider the following two summaries about pentoxifylline, written in 1979 and in 2010 – and then begin contemplating why you are not considering this inexpensive and versatile medication more often.

"... [P]entoxifylline offers a new approach to ameliorate impaired blood flow in ... microvasculature. ... [N]umerous experimental and clinical data ... demonstrate efficacy in ... cerebrovascular insufficiency, senile organic brain syndrome, transient ischemic attacks, cerebral infarctions, ocular and otological circulatory disorders, peripheral angiopathies ... , leg ulcers and other disturbances. ... [T]he efficacy is based on improving local hyperviscosity, hyperaggregability of red cells or platelets,

4

erythrocyte fluidity, and hypercoagulability, resulting in a **better oxygenation of affected tissues**."

R Muller. [1979] [all boldings in this manuscript are added]

"... Pentoxifylline, a synthetic theobromine derivative, is a non-steroidal immunomodulating agent with unique hemorrheologic effects which has been used in a range of infectious, vascular, and inflammatory conditions in adults and children. ... Pentoxifylline has anti-inflammatory properties resulting from inhibition of erythrocyte phosphodiesterase. It lowers blood viscosity and improves microcirculation and tissue perfusion. As a phosphodiesterase inhibitor, **pentoxifylline down-regulates pro-inflammatory cytokines** [cell-communicating glycoprotein hormones] **such as tumor necrosis factor-alpha [TNF-alpha], interleukin-6 [IL-6], and interferon-gamma [IFG].** ... **Pentoxifylline-related significant adverse events are ... very rare.** ..."

E Harris, SM Schulzke, SK Patole. [2010]

Consider the following article's title plus a different article's opening lines – both published in early 2011 – and then contemplate whether your comprehension of this inexpensive and versatile medication might be somewhat out of date:

"**Pentoxifylline (anti-tumor necrosis factor drug)**: effective adjuvant therapy in the control of ocular cicatricial pemphigoid."

MA El Darouti, MA Fakhry Khattab,
RA Hegazy, DA Hafez, HI Gawdat. [2011]

"**As an anti-TNF agent that targets inflammatory process directly, Pentoxifylline** has been investigated for treatment of NASH [non-alcoholic steatohepatitis] in individual studies and pilot trials for years."

W Li, L Zheng, C Sheng, X Cheng, L Qing, S Qu. [2011]

The authors are communicating clearly their belief that pentoxifylline needs to be recharacterized.

A number of recent randomized controlled studies noted the **steroid-sparing effects** of pentoxifylline in pulmonary sarcoidosis, the **proteinuria-reducing effects** of pentoxifylline in kidney disease, the **morbidity-reducing effects** of pentoxifylline in advanced cirrhosis, the **anti-fibrosis effects** of pentoxifylline in connective tissue disease, the **sociability-enhancing effects** of pentoxifylline in autism, the **myocardium-protecting effects** of pentoxifylline in heart surgery, the **analgesic-enhancing effects** of pentoxifylline in nephrolithotomy, and the **mortality-reducing effects** of pentoxifylline in peritonitis. The data are especially strong in regard to renal and hepatic impairment. How many other medications have been demonstrated to have that many uses? How many physicians encounter patients without at least one of these disorders?

The initial understanding was that, as a **synthetic methylxanthine derivative**, pentoxifylline was primarily a **vasodilator** – and much of the earliest research concerned its beneficial effects on cerebral blood flow. Pentoxifylline first received "marketing approval" in the US in 1984, for the "indication" of "intermittent claudication on the basis of chronic occlusive arterial disease of the limbs" – a phrasing that quickly was interpreted to include some aspects of what now is called "restless leg syndrome". Within several years investigators appreciated that pentoxifylline **enhanced red blood cell deformability and slipperiness** – which both allows blood cells to slide down smaller vessels and allows blood cells to resist easy breakage; that is, that pentoxifylline both **reduced ischemia** and **reduced anemia**. By 1989 investigators appreciated that pentoxifylline **functioned as an anti-inflammatory TNF-alpha blocker**, and by 1994 that it **functioned as a non-selective phosphodiesterase inhibitor** [PDE 1-5 but primarily PDE 4], increasing intracellular cyclic adenosine monophosphate (cAMP), a common intracellular second messenger in multiple cell signaling pathways. By 2002 investigators appreciated that pentoxifylline **improved mitochondrial function**, and by 2008 that it **reduced C-reactive protein**. That is, pentoxifylline quickly became known for its ability to **decrease inflammation**, to **increase blood flow**, and generally to **improve physiologic functioning throughout the organism**. As early as 1996 one summary already noted "off-label" use for "psychopathological symptoms

6

in patients with cerebrovascular insufficiency," as well as for "diabetic angiopathies and neuropathies ..., sickle cell thalassemias ..., high altitude sickness, asthenozoospermia ..., and Raynaud's phenomenon." Currently the medication is used widely for renal, hepatic, cardiovascular, and dermatologic conditions – with increasing use for pulmonary, rheumatologic, gynecologic, and oncologic conditions – among others. Citing its use by high-altitude mountain climbers, several athletics websites helpfully comment that pentoxifylline "is not currently banned by any sporting governing body." That is, off-label use is both widespread and growing – with most of the uses relating to **enhancement of blood flow**, to **reduction of inflammation**, or to both.

In late-2014 http://clinicaltrials.gov listed twenty-seven active studies involving pentoxifylline – with the studies running the gamut – from chronic congestive heart failure to biliary atresia, from brachial plexoplasty to cutaneous leishmaniasis, and from brain metastasis to patent ductus arteriosis. Similarly, http://pubchem.gov categorized pentoxifylline as a **phosphodiesterase inhibitor, platelet aggregation inhibitor, radiation-protective agent, vasodilator agent**, and **free radical scavenger** – while noting its action as an **immunomodulator** – but not noting its known functions as **an apoptotic agent** and as **an antiviral**. Few of those on the cutting edge of science would think of this medication as primarily for "intermittent claudication". That is, **pentoxifylline outgrew its original Food and Drug Administration approved marketing "indication" long, long ago**.

Initially distributed as 100 mg tablets, standard pentoxifylline tablets very early became 400 mg and extended-release. The most common dose is 400 mg ER three times per day, although a number of recent regimens advise twice that amount – a total of 2,400 mg per day. While most patients have no side-effects, the most common problem, if there is one, is nausea – and perhaps vomiting – especially with initial or large individual doses; the second most common problem would be mild hypotension. There are only two reports in the medical literature of intentional overdose – and, indeed, the one [1984], concerning ingestion of about 12 to 13 times the common daily dose, documented four-hours worth of nausea and vomiting. The other report [1998], concerning ingestion of about 75 times the common daily dose, noted circulatory collapse. A just published comparison of pentoxifylline with cilostazol, its competitor for treating the FDA "indication" of intermittent claudication [now expanded to "leg pain"], noted that both medications had nausea as an initially potential issue, but that cilostazol also tended to cause headache and palpitations. While **pentoxifylline does not induce cytochrome P450 and does not accumulate following multiple doses**, cilostazol does both; while **pentoxifylline is only 45% protein-bound**, cilostazol is over 95% protein-bound; while **pentoxifylline does not raise vascular endothelial growth factor (VEGF)**, cilostazol does; while **pentoxifylline is not contraindicated in congestive heart failure** – which it helps – cilostazol is. These significant differences taken together make medication interactions, toxicity, and long-term side-effects far less likely with pentoxifylline. **While pentoxifylline itself does not accumulate following multiple doses, it is becoming increasing clear that its therapeutic actions do: the longer it is used, the more the effect.** Generally, pentoxifylline is viewed as benign and quite safe – which is why it is being used in "common" and "double" dose in so many areas of medical practice.

An astounding proportion of the medical literature on pentoxifylline concerns children – even infants. An article published in 1987 was the first of many to explore the use of pentoxifylline to treat progressive sensorineural hearing loss. In 1994 the first of many articles appeared on the use of pentoxifylline to treat neonatal sepsis. That same year an article appeared on the use of relatively high-dose pentoxifylline (1,600 mg/day) to treat childhood cystic fibrosis, and the following year an article appeared on the use of pentoxifylline to treat pediatric cerebral malaria. An article on using pentoxifylline to treat children with severe systemic lupus appeared in 2000, while pediatric articles on treating progressive myopia and chronic lung disease appeared in 2004. The notion of using nebulized pentoxifylline to treat infantile bronchopulmonary dysplasia was introduced in 2006. That is, **age has not been and is not an issue in prescribing pentoxifylline**. This medication **outgrew its primary association with the "intermittent claudication" seen in older**

patients long, long ago.

A common misconception is that pentoxifylline is a "blood thinner" – or that **its ability to make red blood cells more flexible and thus able to squeeze into small spaces** might enhance a risk for bleeding. Actual data demonstrate that bleeding risk is minimal to non-existent and that pentoxifylline **reduces anemia by enhancing red blood cell survivability**. That is, despite continued "warnings" in the Physicians' Desk Reference, other than occasional mild gastritis associated with nausea from introducing the medication too rapidly, **bleeding risk generally has not been and is not a significant issue in prescribing pentoxifylline**.

Another common misconception is that since oral/ topical pentoxifylline, available generically for over a decade, only partially and relatively briefly reduces TNF-alpha that must make it less desirable clinically than newer injectable long-acting monoclonal antibodies [eg, infliximab, adalimumab, etc], backed by astounding advertising budgets, that almost completely block TNF-alpha. Such is not necessarily the case. **TNF-alpha** [cachectin], produced primarily by [bone marrow] macrophages/ monocytes, along with TNF-beta [lymphotoxin], produced primarily by [thymus] T cells, **supports normal immune function when it is present in the right amount**. Inflammation problems arise when TNF-alpha is secreted in excess and infection problems arise when it is blocked in excess. While the phrase "TNF-alpha blocker" is commonly used, it would be more correct to consider that **pentoxifylline is an inhibitor of cytokine synthesis rather than an anti-cytokine per se**. While the more potent monoclonal antibody immunomodulators either directly block circulating TNF-alpha or inhibit TNF-alpha converting enzyme [TACE] from freeing up membrane-bound TNF-alpha, pentoxifylline works earlier in the sequence – intracellularly – selectively reducing messenger ribonucleic acid [mRNA] coding for the production of TNF-alpha – which is similar in manner to one way in which anti-inflammatory corticosteroids function. That is, as with many other physiologic situations, **regulation versus dysregulation is the clinical issue** rather than stimulation versus eradication, and **mimicking natural**

pathways appears to be less disruptive. Just as there has been a body of research exploring the use of pentoxifylline to reduce clinical steroid use, now there is developing a body of research exploring the use of pentoxifylline to reduce monoclonal antibody use. As one might expect, the race is now on to develop patentable delivery systems for the off-patent pentoxifylline – especially delivery systems that could provide large doses to the brain over a long span of hours, as data suggest would be needed for the practical treatment of senile dementia ["Alzheimer's disease"].

Yet another common misconception is that since oral/ topical pentoxifylline is a non-selective phosphodiesterase [PDE] inhibitor – reducing PDEs 1 through 5 but mostly PDE 4 – that must make it and related molecules less desirable than newer more potent and selective PDEs. Once again, such is not necessarily the case. PDE-1 inhibition primarily induces cerebral, cardiac, and pulmonary vasorelaxation; PDE-2 inhibition primarily decreases aldosterone secretion, decreases inflammation of internal organ microvessels, improves platelet and monocyte adhesion, plus may both dampen anxiety and enhance memory; PDE-3 inhibition primarily enhances the force and speed of smooth muscle contraction while also enhancing smooth muscle relaxation and antagonizing platelet aggregation; PDE-5 inhibition primarily also enhances smooth muscle relaxation. **While a main action of pentoxifylline is PDE-4 inhibition, suppressing the release of inflammatory mediators, the fact that it works synergistically with a number of other areas of PDE inhibition appears to render the net effect superior to many other more selective PDE inhibitors.** That is, again, a smoother and broader approach may be preferable to a more dramatic and focused one. While the race is still on to develop patentable products, it appears that one strategy may well be to pair a more selective and potent PDE inhibitor with a non-selective one such as pentoxifylline.

One has to be struck by the admirable safety profile of pentoxifylline – and by the magnitude of articles written by pediatricians and surgeons. Both of these groups of specialists have recognized the immune modulating aspects of pentoxifylline, and now psychiatrists are poised to move the story forward. **Pentoxifylline most clearly and** cleanly down-regulates TNF-alpha, and, in a somewhat more complex manner down-regulates IL-6 – both of these being pro-inflammatory cytokines. In just happens that these are the same two cytokines now most commonly associated with depression – especially with suicidal behavior – and apparently with other affective and cognitive disorders, such as anxiety, bipolar disorder, schizophrenia, Alzheimer's, and autism – that is, an array of neuropsychiatric conditions. Several major reviews of the associations between inflammation and depression have been published since 2008, the focus thus far being on demonstrating shifts in TNF-alpha, IL-6, and other inflammatory cytokine levels during treatment or on noting incidental reductions in depression during anti-cytokine treatment of non-psychiatric disorders. Several so-called "antidepressants" and "antipsychotics" have anti-inflammatory capacity, but – thus far – there are no known head-to-head comparisons with pentoxifylline.

While specifically psychiatric literature on the use of pentoxifylline is sparse, one of the oldest articles is the most intriguing. An observational study published in 1979, using only 300 mg per day of pentoxifylline for 7 weeks, in 26 cognitively-impaired patients ranging in age from 56 to 89 years old, noted dramatic improvements in vertigo, headache, insomnia, memory, mental drive, concentration, fatigue, motivation, physical endurance, sociability, negativity, and apathy. The statistics are crude but still notable: 23% had excellent results, another 26% had good results, and another 30% had at least some degree of global improvement. A similar but double-blinded study also published in 1979, using 1,200 mg per day of pentoxifylline for 8 weeks, in 29 cognitively-impaired geriatric patients, noted significant improvements in insomnia, sociability, and global performance on psychometric testing. A review updated in early 2010 noted that, in a double-blinded, placebo-controlled, multicenter study, pentoxifylline indeed produced significant cognitive improvement in multi-infarct patients.

Most recent research on the cognitive and affective effects of pentoxifylline has been conducted with mice – which may reflect the paucity of funding for investigations using an off-patent medication. For the record, let it be noted that pentoxifylline is anxiolytic and memory enhancing in mice. Let it also be noted that a patentable PDE-4 inhibitor demonstrated definite antipsychotic and antidepressant action but had side-effect issues. Both **pentoxifylline** and propentofylline – a structural analogue of pentoxifylline – have been shown to have **direct effect on glial tissue**, and are being investigated for possible use in the treatment of schizophrenia and **chronic – especially neuropathic – pain syndromes**. Given the recent surge of research in humans linking pentoxifylline with cytokine reduction, and linking cytokine reduction with antidepressant activity –including anti-suicide activity – along with the parallel research in humans on the immune modulating properties of several so-called "antidepressants" and "antipsychotics" – one might anticipate an upcoming direct investigation of the antidepressant/ anti-suicidal/ anxiolytic/ antipsychotic/ analgesic potential of pentoxifylline – as soon as pharmaceutical companies figure out how to tweak the molecule and thus make such research more cost-effective.

As a leading investigator of this medication, Professor Whitehouse, has commented, pentoxifylline almost became, quite inappropriately, an "orphan drug". "Re-focusing on patient needs, rather than drug company profits, would certainly assist serious re-evaluation of PTX [pentoxifylline] … ." As a much-cited healthcare economics article on "Bayesian value-of-information-analysis" specifically demonstrated in regard to pentoxifylline, once it is known to be useful in a condition the "estimate of uncertainty surrounding the cost effectiveness" of adding it suggests that there is little room for argument. To summarize, pentoxifylline appears to "enhance survivability" and improve physiologic functioning in a wide variety of clinical situations. The list of mechanisms involved continues to grow in this very active area of biomedical research. In the meantime, on a practical basis, when might you want to consider the prescription of the venerable pentoxifylline, at least in a trial dose of one 400 mg ER tablet with food? Surely a great number of patients have one or more of the many, many conditions for which pentoxifylline has been found to be clean, safe, and effective.

While pentoxifylline shares some properties with other xanthines

– especially its precursor "pentifylline" and its main metabolite "lisofylline" – pentoxifylline stands out for its balance of positive physiologic actions.

CAFFEINE $C_8H_{10}N_4O_2$
1,3,7-trimethylxanthine

THEOPHYLLINE $C_7H_8N_4O_2$
3,7-dimethylxanthine [isomer of theobromine]

THEOBROMINE $C_7H_8N_4O_2$
3,7-dimethylxanthine [isomer of theophylline]

PENTIFYLLINE $C_{13}H_{20}N_4O_2$
1-hexyl-3,7-dimethylxanthine
very potent; a precursor of pentoxifylline in discovery & structure; a synthetic mixture of theobromine & hexyl halide.

PENTOXIFYLLINE $\mathbf{C_{13}H_{18}N_4O_3}$
1-(5-oxohexyl)-3,7-dimethylxanthine
a metabolite of pentifylline; a precursor & sometime metabolite of lisofylline & hydroxypentoxifylline; a synthetic derivative of theobromine.

LISOFYLLINE $C_{13}H_{20}N_4O_3$
1-(5-R-hydroxyhexyl)-3,7-dimethylxanthine
a reversible metabolite ["R-M1"] & therefore sometime precursor of pentoxifylline.

PROPENTOFYLLINE $C_{15}H_{22}N_4O_3$
1-(5-oxohexyl)-3-methyl-7-propylxanthine
a structural analogue of pentoxifylline.

HYDROXYPROPENTOFYLLINE $C_{15}H_{22}N_4O_4$
1-(5-hydroxyhexyl)-3,5-dimethyl-7 propylxanthin
a metabolite of propentofylline.

DENBUFYLLINE $C_{16}H_{24}N_4O_3$
7-acetonyl-1,3-dibutylxanthine
very potent; analogue of pentoxifylline.

HYDROXYPENTOXIFYLLINE $C_{13}H_{20}N_4O_3$
1-(5-S-hydroxyhexyl)-3,7-dimethylxanthine
very potent; a reversible metabolite ["S-M1"] & therefore sometime precursor of pentoxifylline.

HYDROXYPENTOXIFYLLINE D6 $C_{13}H_{14}D_6N_4O_3$
1-(5-S-hydroxyhexyl)-3,7-dimethylxanthine-D6
"CTP-499"; a deuterated analogue of the "S-M1" metabolite of pentoxifylline, said to have a longer half-life.

DOXOFYLLINE $C_{11}H_{14}N_4O_4$
1-(3-carboxypropyl)-3,7-dimethylxanthine
an irreversible metabolite ["M-5"] of pentoxifylline.

The increasing research interest in pentoxifylline and related compounds cannot be ignored. The following table, based on data derived from www.PubMed.gov, indicates the number of medical articles per year published on pentoxifylline and its "relatives" in sequential 5-year periods. The potent precursor pentifylline (marketed in combination with niacinamide) was allowed to languish after it went off patent; the similarly potent doxofylline (M-5 metabolite of pentoxifylline) is attracting more attention, especially as an anti-inflammatory bronchodilator.

	human-pentox	non-human-pentox	**TOTAL-PENTOX**	total- penti-, liso-, propentox-, hydroxypropentox-,denbu-, doxofylline; (including penti+niacinamide)	**TOTAL-ALL ARTICLES RELATING TO PENTOXIFYLLINE**
2014	32	**105**	137	11	**148**
2013	42	70	112	**19**	131
2012	**91**	**83**	**174**	**19**	**193**
2011	68	34	102	15	117
2006-10	**404**	27	**676**	22	**698**
2001-05	285	**136**	421	28	449
1996-00	133	77	210	**55**	265
1991-95	146	74	220	45	265
1986-90	88	119	207	32	239
1981-85	62	18	80	4	84
1976-80	103	42	145	25	170
1971-75	1	3	4	8	12

Interestingly enough, if one repeats the analysis looking only at the 120 journals that PubMed historically has segregated as its "core clinical journals" collection, an entirely different view emerges – one of interest in pentoxifylline and related compounds peaking during the 5-year period of 1996-2000 and then diminishing across the board. Stated another way, **after pentoxifylline went off-patent in the United States in 1998 the supposedly more prestigious journals lost interest – while the generally non-Anglo-American journals retained or gained interest**, as conveyed in the numbers noted above in contrast to those noted below. One has to wonder if this skewed publication pattern occurs concerning other medications – that certain editors, authors, and readers become less interested once a medication is not being promoted by a pharmaceutical company, while certain other editors, authors, and readers become more interested once the price of a medication is no longer supported by a patent. [Another observation, if one looks at the specifically mentioned agents in the articles: as the broader population of journals began showing an increased interest in recent years in pentoxifylline, the "core clinical journals" began showing an increased interest in propentofylline, which currently is marketed only as a veterinary medication.]

	human-pentox	non-human-pentox	TOTAL-PENTOX	total- penti-, liso-, propentox-, hydroxypropentox-,denbu-, doxofylline; (including penti+niacinamide)	TOTAL-ALL ARTICLES RELATING TO PENTOXIFYLLINE
2014	3	3	6	0	0
2013	6	1	7	19	26
2012	23	18	41	2	43
2011	63	30	93	14	107
2006-10	30	22	52	4	56
2001-05	56	34	90	9	99
1996-00	87	46	133	9	142
1991-95	66	58	122	1	123
1986-90	36	38	74	1	75
1981-85	15	1	16	0	16
1976-80	4	1	5	0	5
1971-75	0	0	0	0	0

The depth and breadth of research on pentoxifylline – compared to the relative infrequency of its current use – is astounding.

PENTOXIFYLLINE:

A VERSATILE OFF-PATENT MEDICINE BEST NOT OVERLOOKED

> BIBLIOGRAPHY, PRIMARILY OF ABSTRACTS OF HUMAN STUDIES
*** NOTE ***

**Many of the following references easily
could have been placed in more than one category.**
First consult the most likely category,
then consider consulting the next most likely category.

Much is to be gained from scanning virtually all of the following
references, which are arranged in reverse chronological order.

The vast majority of these references concern research in humans –
but an occasional reference concerns research in non-humans
(eg, rats, mice, etc) if the findings seemed especially important.

An occasional reference will not mention pentoxifylline *per se* but
will be relevant to the overall discussion of its actions.

ADVANCES IN DELIVERY SYSTEMS & TWEAKING OF THE MOLECULE

Pentoxifylline and propentofylline both are "off patent," so, of course, the race is on to investigate their metabolites, synergistic combinations, and improved means of delivery. **Hydroxypentoxifylline-D6** as of November 2014 was being readied for phase 3 clinical trials for diabetic nephropathy, as a once-a-day **anti-inflammatory, anti-oxidant, anti-fibrotic agent**, while having only one publication on the entity listed in PubMed. A **fixed combination of pentoxifylline plus N-acetylcysteine** was expected to enter phase 1 clinical trials for pulmonary fibrosis in the second quarter of 2012, as a once-a-day **anti-inflammatory, anti-oxidant, anti-fibrotic, anti-neutrophil sequestrator,** and pan-phosphodiesterase inhibitor, without having any publications on the entity listed in PubMed.

The abstracts listed below suggest the magnitude of investigation in this area – toward producing a patentable version of pentoxifylline – even though many patients world-wide could be served adequately by the original molecular formulations.

Nagaich U, Bharti C, Pal AK, Gulati N. "Preparation and evaluation of pentoxifylline loaded **chewable tablet for the treatment of peripheral vascular diseases**." Der Pharmacia Lettre, 2014;6(1):58-64.

Labib GS, Farid RM. "Osteogenic effect of locally applied Pentoxyfilline gel: in vitro and in vivo evaluations." Drug Deliv. 2014 Feb 20; "… to formulate **Pentoxyfylline drug (PTX) as a local bioadhesive Carbopol**

(Cbp) based gel for the aid of bone induction around an endosseus oral implant. ... Two concentrations of 1% and 3% Cbp containing 1% PTX were prepared. ... In vivo experimental results in rabbits have shown significant difference in bone depth induction of 3% and 1% Cbp gels with the formation of strong organized bone over the control group. **Local administration of Pentoxifylline could be regarded as a valid approach in the management of osseointegration.**"

Nisi A, Panfili M, De Rosa G, Boffa G, Groppa F, Gusella M, Padrini R. "Pharmacokinetics of pentoxifylline and its main metabolites in patients with different degrees of heart failure following a single dose of a modified-release formulation." J Clin Pharmacol. 2013 Jan;53(1):51-7; "...The time courses of PTX [pentoxifylline], [and its 3 metabolites] M1, M4, and M5 plasma levels were determined after oral administration of **a [new] sustained-release 600-mg tablet ... [for] patients with severe CHF [congestive heart failure]** compared with moderate CHF ...."

Mohamed T, Osman W, Tin G, Rao PP. "Selective inhibition of human acetylcholinesterase by xanthine derivatives: In vitro inhibition and molecular modeling investigations." Bioorg Med Chem Lett. 2013 Aug 1;23(15):4336-41; "... **pentoxifylline and propentofylline are able to bind to both the catalytic site and peripheral anionic site [of acetylcholinesterase (AChE)]** due to their increased bulk/size, thereby exhibiting superior AChE inhibition relative to caffeine. ..."

Kim H, Kim Y, Guk K, Yoo D, Lim H, Kang G, Lee D. "Fully biodegradable and cationic poly(amino oxalate) particles for the treatment of acetaminophen-induced acute liver failure." Int J Pharm. 2012 Sep 15;434(1-2):243-50; "... Poly(amino oxalate) (PAOX) is a new family of fully biodegradable polymer that possesses tertiary amine groups in its backbone and has rapid hydrolytic degradation. ... The high therapeutic efficacy of **PTX[pentoxifylline]-loaded PAOX particles for ALF [acute liver failure]** treatment [in a mouse model] may be attributed to the unique properties of PAOX particles, which **can target passively liver, stimulate cellular uptake and trigger a colloid osmotic disruption of the phagosome to release encapsulated PTX into the cytosol. ...**"

Gupta Vishnu D. "Chemical stability of pentoxifylline in a topical cream." Int J Pharmaceutical Compound. Jan/Feb 2012;16(1):80-81; "**...**The **topical [pentoxifylline] cream** was stable for at least 62 days when stored in white opaque ointment jars (plastic) at room temperature. ..."

Lin HY, Yeh CT. "Genipin-crosslinked chitosan scaffolds and its efficacy in releasing anti-inflammatory medicine." Biomed Mater Eng. 2012 Jan 1;22(5):321-32; "... In vitro tests showed that **when PTX [pentoxifylline] was released more slowly from crosslinked scaffolds, PTX became more effective in suppressing macrophage cells from releasing IL-6 and TNF-α.**"

Yougbare I, Morin C, Senouvo FY, Sirois C, Albadine R, Lugnier C, Rousseau E. "NCS 613, **a potent and specific PDE4 inhibitor**, displays anti-inflammatory effects on human lung tissues." Am J Physiol Lung Cell Mol Physiol. 2011 Oct;301(4):L441-50; "... Pharmacological treatments with NCS 613 significantly decreased PDE4 activity and reduced IκBα degradation in cultured parenchyma, both of which are usually correlated with a lower inflammation status. Moreover, NCS 613 pretreatment potentiated isoproterenol-induced relaxations in human distal bronchi, while reducing TNF-α-induced hyper-responsiveness in cultured bronchi, as assessed in the presence of methacholine, U-46619, or histamine. ... In conclusion, **specific PDE4 inhibitors, such as NCS 613, may represent an alternative and isoform-specific approach toward reducing human lung inflammation and airway overreactivity.**"

Sant VP, Nagarsenker MS. "Synthesis of monomethoxypoly-ethyleneglycol-cholesteryl ester and effect of its incorporation in liposomes." AAPS Pharm Sci Tech. 2011 Aug 19; "... Conventional and **PEG-CH [monomethoxypolyethyleneglycol-5000 cholesteryl ester] containing pentoxyfylline liposomes** did not show any signs of pentoxyfylline degradation when stored at 4°C for 3 months."

Abbar JC, Malode SJ, Nandibewoor ST. "Electrochemical determination of a hemorheologic drug, pentoxifylline at a multi-walled carbon nanotube paste electrode." Bioelectrochemistry. 2011 Jul 5; "**The electrochemical oxidation of … pentoxifylline was investigated at a multi-walled carbon nanotubes-paraffin oil paste electrode using cyclic and differential pulse voltammetry**. The oxidation process was irreversible over the pH range studied and exhibited an adsorption-controlled behavior. … This method can also be employed in quality control and routine determination of drugs in pharmaceutical formulations."

Alarfaj N, El-Tohamy M. "New validated potentiometric determination of vasodilator pentoxifylline in its pharmaceutical formulations and biological fluids." J Chinese Chem Soc (Taipei) 2011 Jun 3;58(4); http://proj3.sinica.edu.tw/~chem/servxx6/files/paper_13776_1307091100 .pdf "The pentoxifylline-selective electrodes based on pentoxifylline-phosphotungstate ion association in a PVC [polyvinylchloride] matrix exhibited useful analytical characteristics for the determination of pentoxifylline in pure form, pharmaceutical formulations and biological fluids. … Moreover, the method is simple, easy to operate and inexpensive making it **an excellent tool for the routine determination of pentoxifylline in quality control laboratories**."

Walczak M, Kozaczek E, Szymura-Oleksiak J, Pękala E. "Application of liquid chromatography-tandem mass spectrometry method for the simultaneous quantitative analysis of propentofylline and its chiral metabolite M1 in rats." Biomed Chromatogr. 2011 Mar;25(3):381-90; "A sensitive and selective liquid chromatographic-electrospray ionization mass spectrometric method for the simultaneous determination of propentofylline and enantiomers of its active metabolite M1 [lisofylline] in rat serum, cortex and hippocampus was developed and validated according to GLP [good laboratory practice] procedures. … **The established LC/ESI-MS/MS [chromatography electrospray ionization tandem mass spectrometry] method has been successfully applied to an initial pharmacokinetic study of propentofylline and also to assessment of distribution of parent drug and enantiomers of its pharmacologically active metabolite M1 to cortex and hippocampus** after intravenous administration of propentofylline to rats at a dose of 5 mg/kg."

Al-Zoubi N, Kachrimanis K, Younis K, Malamataris S. "Optimization of extended-release hydrophilic matrix tablets by support vector regression." Drug Dev Ind Pharm. 2011 Jan;37(1):80-7. [re "the **optimization of extended release from swellable hydrophilic pentoxifylline matrix-tablets"**]

Pirvu CD, Ortan A, Hirjau M, Prisada R, Lupuleasa D, Bogdan A. "Studies concerning **the optimization of the pentoxifylline encapsulation.**" Romanian Biotech Letters. 2011:16(1) supplement.

Sora DI, Cristea E, Albu F, David V, Medvedovici A. "Bioanalysis of pentoxifylline and related metabolites in plasma samples through LC-MS/MS." Biomed Chromatogr. 2010 Jun;24(6):663-74; "... Analytical aspects related to **the assay of pentoxifylline (PTX), lisofylline (M1) and carboxypropyl dimethylxanthine (M5) metabolites** are discussed through comparison of two alternative analytical methods based on liquid chromatography separation and atmospheric pressure electrospray ionization tandem mass spectrometry detection. ... Both analytical methods were fully validated and used **to assess bioequivalence between a prolonged release generic formulation and the reference product, under multidose and single dose approaches.**"

Varshosaz J, Minayian M, E. Moazen E. (2010): "**Enhancement of oral bioavailability of pentoxifylline by solid lipid nanoparticles.**" J Liposome Res. 2010;20(2):115-1123.

Shivhare UD, Ambulkar DU, Mathur VB, Bhusari KP, Godbole MD (2009): "**Formulation and evaluation of pentoxifylline liposome.**" Digest J Nanomaterials Biostructures. 2009;4(4):857-862.

Pekala E, Kochan M, Carnell AJ. "Microbial transformation of hydroxy metabolites of 1-oxohexyl derivatives of theobromine by Cunninghamella echinulata NRRL 1384." Lett Appl Microbiol. 2009 Jan;48(1):19-24; "...**The biotransformation of pentoxifylline (PTX), propentofylline (PPT) and their racemic hydroxy metabolites ((+/-)-OHPTX and (+/-**

)-OHPPT) by using the fungus **Cunninghamella echinulata NRRL 1384**. ...The bioconversion of (+/-)-OHPTX gave an (R)-enantiomer (LSF-lisofylline) with a higher enantiopurity (maximum approximately 93% ee) compared to the bioconversion of (+/-)-OHPPT, when the maximum ee value for (R)-OHPPT was recorded at 83%. ... The conversion of (+/-)-OHPTX and (+/-)-OHPPT using Cunninghamella echinulata ... may be recommended as an alternative ... ."

Tamizharasi S, Rathi JC, Rathi V. (2008): "Formulation and evaluation of **pentoxifylline-loaded poly(ε-caprolactone) microspheres.**" Indian J Pharm Sci. 2008;70(3):333-337.

Martin, L, Wilson CG, Koosha F, Uchegbu IF "**Sustained buccal delivery of the hydrophobic drug denbufylline using physically cross-linked palmitoyl glycol chitosan hydrogels.**" European J Pharmaceutics Biopharmaceutics. 2003 Jan;55(1):35-45

Kwon OS, Chung YB, Kim MH, Hahn HG, Rhee HK, Ryu JC. "**Pharmacokinetics of propentofylline and the quantitation of its metabolite hydroxypropentofylline in human volunteers.**" Arch Pharm Res. 1998 Dec;21(6):698-702.

GENERAL COMMENTS, including Formulations, High Dosing,
      Safety Profile (including Research in Infants), Vascular Effects,
      Anti-Inflammatory Effects (plus Anti-Cytokine Crisis Effects),
      Immune Modulating Effects, & Steroid-Sparing Properties

The abstracts listed below outline the progressive appreciation historically of what pentoxifylline and its analogues can do – safely and effectively.

Cakmak SK, Cakmak A, Gönül M, Kılıç A, Gül U. "Pentoxifyllıne use in dermatology." Inflamm Allergy Drug Targets. 2012 Dec 1;11(6):422-32; "...Novel **immunomodulatory properties of pentoxifylline** have been reported including the **down regulation of tumour necrosis factor-α**

synthesis and other inflammatory cytokines. Studies have shown that pentoxifylline might be **efficacious in a wide spectrum of skin diseases.** ..."

Ibelgaufts H. "Pentoxifylline." COPE/ Cytokines & Cells Online Pathfinder Encyclopaedia. "Spring/Summer 2010 Ed." http://www.copewithcytokines.de/cope.cgi?key=Pentoxifylline [a comprehensive summary of **the complex immunomodulating effects of pentoxifylline**]; "reduces the levels of circulating TNF and IL6"; **"reduces the amounts of circulating TNF without influencing the endogenous synthesis of other Interleukins."**

de Albuquerque RM, Virgini-Magalhães CE, Lencastre Sicuro F, Bottino DA, Bouskela E. "Effects of cilostazol and pentoxifylline on forearm reactive hyperemia response, lipid profile, oxidative stress, and inflammatory markers in patients with intermittent claudication." Angiology. 2008 Oct-Nov;59(5):549-58; **"pentoxifylline reduced C-reactive protein level** and increased maximal walking distance in total and nonsmoking groups."

Deree J, Lall R, Melbostad H, Loomis W, Hoyt DB, Coimbra R. "Pentoxifylline attenuates stored blood-induced inflammation: A new perspective on an old problem." Surgery. 2006 Aug;140(2):186-91; "... PTX [pentoxifylline] administration resulted in a 106% decrease in TNF-alpha .... **PTX [pentoxifylline] downregulates ... TNF-alpha expression in supernatant-induced whole blood.** Because blood transfusion can contribute to inflammatory injury, the adjunctive use of PTX may have therapeutic potential."

Iglesias C, Claxton K. "Comprehensive decision analytic modeling and Baysesian value of information analysis: the case of pentoxifylline in the treatment of chronic venous leg ulcers." Pharmacoeconomics. 2006;24(5):465-78. [There is a competing article by another team of health economists: Guest JF, Davie AM, Clegg JP. "Cost effectiveness of cilostazol compared with naftidrofuryl and pentoxifylline in the treatment of intermittent claudication in the UK." Curr Med Res Opin. 2005

Jun;21(6):817-26; the considerably more expensive cilostazol/ Pletal, like pentoxifylline/ Trental, is available in the US, but the even more expensive naftidrofuryl / Dusodril is not. The argument goes on: the UK National Institute for Health and Clinical Excellence commissioned a major study, not yet seen, of "the incremental cost effectiveness" of "Cilostazol, naftidrofuryl oxalate, pentoxifylline and inositol nicotinate for the treatment of intermittent claudication in people with peripheral arterial disease." This could get very interesting – with a lot of money at stake – because all four medications (the latter one – "no flush" niacin – being "dirt cheap") are under investigation for use in Alzheimer's disease.]

O'Neil MJ, ed. "Phosphodiesterase Inhibitors." The Merck Index: An Encyclopedia of Chemicals, Drugs, and Biologicals, 14th ed. (Whitehouse Station, NJ, 2006).

Bender AT, Beavo JA. "Cyclic nucleotide phosphodiesterases: molecular regulation to clinical use." Pharmacol. Rev. 2006 Sep;58(3): 488–520 [detailed review of the PDE families]; http://pharmrev.aspetjournals.org/content/58/3/488.long#ref-17

Whitehouse MW. "Anti-TNF-α therapy for chronic inflammation: reconsidering pentoxifylline as an alternative to therapeutic protein drugs." Inflammopharmacology. 2004;12(3):223-7, pp.223, 226 [highlights: Strieter RM, Remick DG, Ward PA, Spengler RN, Lynch JP 3rd, Larrick J, Kunkel SL. "Cellular and molecular regulation of tumor necrosis factor-alpha production by pentoxifylline." Biochem Biophys Res Commun. 1988 Sep 30;155(3):1230-6; this short but key article by Whitehouse, a foremost authority on anti-inflammation, is available free at both http://www.springerlink.com/content/b6ca36b55c6e9f44 and http://www.docstoc.com/docs/48065853/Points-of-View-Anti-TNF-therapy-for-chronic-inflammation; see also the editorial comment on this article: Rainsford KD. "New combinations of anti-inflammatories for therapy of arthritic, neurological and malignant diseases." Inflammopharmacology. 2004;12(3):211-3 – also available free on the web at http://www.springerlink.com/content/81c05df8c8df0277/

Park E, Schuller-Levis G, Park SY, Jia JH, Levis WR. "Pentoxifylline downregulates nitric oxide and tumor necrosis factor-alpha induced by mycobacterial lipoarabinomannan in a macrophage cell line." Int J Lepr Other Mycobact Dis. 2001 Sep;69(3):225-33; "... **Pentoxifylline (PTX) .... also showed moderate inhibition of NO [nitric oxide]** at the product level as well as translation of iNOS [inducible nitric oxide synthase]."

Beshay E, Croze F, Prud'homme GJ. "The phosphodiesterase inhibitors pentoxifylline and rolipram suppress macrophage activation and nitric oxide production in vitro and in vivo." Clin Immunol. 2001 Feb;98(2):272-9; "...**The inhibition of NO production of macrophages by ... PTX [pentoxifylline] could be beneficial in NO [nitric oxide]-mediated inflammatory and/or autoimmune disorders.**"

Teixeira MM, Gristwood RW, Cooper N, Hellewell PG. "Phosphodiesterase (PDE)4 inhibitors: anti-inflammatory drugs of the future?" Trends Pharmacol Sci. 1997 May;18(5):164-71; "Phosphodiesterase type 4 (PDE4) plays a major role in modulating the activity of virtually all cells involved in the inflammatory process. **Inhibitors of this enzyme family display impressive anti-inflammatory and disease-modifying effects in a variety of experimental models. ...**"

Kamphuis J, Smits P, Thien T. "Vascular effects of pentoxifylline in humans." J Cardiovasc Pharmacol. 1994 Oct;24(4):648-54; "Our data further suggest that pentoxifylline-induced vasodilation is not mediated by adenosine receptor stimulation, but may result from inhibition of the enzyme phosphodiesterase (PDE)" [**more clearly appreciated pentoxifylline as a phosphodiesterase inhibitor**].

VA National Acquisition Center. "Notice of intent to procure a bundled contract [Department of Veterans Affairs/ Department of Defense]: Request for Proposal (RFP) 797-NC-05-0049 for Pentoxifylline Tablets 400 mg, SA"; ftp://ftp.fbo.gov/FBOFeed20050819

Olin BR, Hebel SK, editors. "Pentoxifylline." Drug Facts and Comparisons: 1996 edition. St. Louis: Facts and Comparisons/ Wolters

Kluwer, 1996; pp.348-9; p.348.

Ernst E. ["20 years pentoxifylline: a part of recent angiology history."] [article in German; abstract in English is per www.pubmed.gov] Wien Med Wochenschr. 1992;142(19):433-7.

Müller R. "Pentoxifylline – a biomedical profile." J Med. 1979;10(5):307-29.

Stefanovich V. "Effect of 3,7-dimethyl-1-(5-oxo-hexyl)xanthine [pentoxifylline] and 1-hexyl-3,7-dimethyl xanthine [pentifylline] on cyclic AMP phosphodiesterase of the human umbilical cord vessels." Res Commun Chem Pathol Pharmacol. 1973 May;5(3):655-62 [via investigations of adenosine perhaps **first appreciated pentoxifylline and its precursor as phosphodiesterase inhibitors**; he went on to appreciate **the neuropsychiatric potential**: Stefanovich V, John JP. "Influence of pentifylline on brain metabolism of normal and anoxic rats." Arzneimittelforschung. 1978;28(11):2097-9].

Clark IA. "How TNF was recognized as a key mechanism of disease." Cytokine Growth Factor Rev. 2007 Jun-Aug;18(3-4):335-43; "the origins of the insight that excess production of pro-inflammatory cytokines caused a constellation of changes that contribute to pathophysiology of disease. This connection was made following the original 1975 TNF (tumor necrosis factor) publication from New York describing how activated macrophages kill tumors. The study caught the eye of a group in London who were trying to understand how the same in vivo macrophage activation would protect mice against the erythrocytic protozoan parasites that cause malaria and babesiosis. Based on collaborative research between these two groups, it was argued in 1981 that TNF and related cytokines initiated events that caused pathology, as well as parasite death within red cells in these infectious diseases. This proved to be a key conceptual advance. It was also argued that the pathology of bacterial sepsis logically had TNF origins. Once TNF was cloned in 1985, allowing its specific analysis in serum and neutralization in vivo, the involvement of this cytokine in infectious disease pathology was pursued by a number of groups. Some researchers found that once 'their' cytokine was cloned and sequenced, they had been unwittingly expanding knowledge on TNF for several years. ... **With its implication as the master regulator of other inflammatory cytokines in the synovial membrane, TNF has also become the major cytokine in the pathogenesis of chronic inflammatory disease. ..."**

Tsokos GC, Atkins JL. Combat medicine: basic and clinical research in military, trauma, and emergency medicine. NY: Humana Press, 2003; pp.77, 81, 118, 121, 129, 329, 344, 349, 424.

Burnouf C, Pruniaux MP. "Recent advances in PDE4 inhibitors as immunoregulators and anti-inflammatory drugs." Curr Pharm Des. 2002;8(14):1255-96; "... the type 4 phosphodiesterase (PDE4) is a cAMP-specific enzyme localized in airway smooth muscle cells as well as in immune and inflammatory cells. The PDE4 activity is associated with a wide variety of diseases some of which have been related to an inflammatory state, (e.g. asthma, chronic obstructive pulmonary disease (COPD), rheumatoid arthritis (RA)) while others have recently been connected to autoimmune pathology. ... This review highlights the recent data of the most advanced clinical candidates, the design and structure activity relationships of the recent structural series reported in the literature over the last two years, as well as recent advances in **the multiple therapeutic indications of PDE4 inhibitors** (a review with 375 references)."

Neuner P, Klosner G, Schauer E, Pourmojib M, Macheiner W, Grünwald C, Knobler R, Schwarz A, Luger TA, and Schwarz T. "Pentoxifylline in vivo down-regulates the release of IL-1 beta, IL-6, IL-8 and tumour necrosis factor-alpha by human peripheral blood mononuclear cells." Immunology. 1994 October; 83(2): 262–267; "incubated in vitro with PTX [pentoxifylline] for 48 hr. Under these conditions, only TNF-alpha was found to be reduced"; "However, when PBMC [peripheral blood mononuclear cells] were **incubated with PTX for 24 hr**, PTX removed thereafter by medium change and cells further cultured, the production **not only of TNF-alpha but also of IL-1 beta, IL-6 and IL-8 was reduced,** demonstrating that **PTX exerts diverse (inhibitory) effects on cytokine release** by PBMC."

Zabel P, Wolter DT, Schönharting MM, Schade UF. "Oxpentifylline in endotoxaemia." Lancet. 1989 Dec 23-30;2(8678-8679):1474-7; "oxpentifylline blocks the endotoxin-induced synthesis of TNF [tumor necrosis factor] in man" [part of **the discovery that pentoxifylline rather than being a "blocker" per se actually is a "TNF-alpha synthesis inhibitor"**].

Sullivan GW, Carper HT, Novick WJ Jr, Mandell GL. "Inhibition of the inflammatory action of interleukin-1 and tumor necrosis factor (alpha) on neutrophil function by pentoxifylline." Infect Immun. 1988 Jul;56(7):1722-9; "...By blocking the inflammatory action of interleukin-1 and tumor necrosis factor on neutrophils, pentoxifylline may diminish the tissue damage caused by neutrophils in such conditions as septic shock, adult respiratory distress syndrome, cardiopulmonary bypass lung damage, and myocardial reperfusion injury." [part of **the discovery that pentoxifylline acts like a "TNF-alpha blocker"**]

El Darouti MA, Fakhry Khattab MA, Hegazy RA, Hafez DA, Gawdat HI. "Pentoxifylline (anti-tumor necrosis factor drug): effective adjuvant therapy in the control of ocular cicatricial pemphigoid." Eur J Ophthalmol. 2011 Jan 28; [30 patients divided into 2 groups; 20 controls] "... The study illustrates that **the addition of [intravenous] pentoxifylline to pulse steroid cyclophosphamide therapy is an effective, safe, and economical method in controlling OCP [ocular cicatricial pemphigoid] through directly reducing TNF-a levels**, with long periods of remission as detected in our 18-month follow-up period."

Park MK, Fontana Jr, Babaali H, Gilbert-McClain LI, Stylianou M, Joo J, Moss J, Manganiello VC. "Steroid-sparing effects of pentoxifylline in pulmonary sarcoidosis." Sarcoidosis Vasc Diffuse Lung Dis. 2009 Jul;26(2):121-31; "**The observed relative risk reduction for flares associated with POF [pentoxifylline] treatment was 54.9% ... and the absolute risk reduction was 50.6%** .... Compared to placebo treatment, in the POF group, the mean prednisone dose was lower at 8 and 10 months … , and **there was a trend towards less prednisone usage over the entire study period** … , as determined by cumulative change analysis."

Marino WD. "Combined pentoxifylline and doxycycline as a steroid-sparing adjuvant regimen in sarcoidosis." American College of Chest Physicians session. 2008 OCT 28; presentation. http://meeting.chestpubs.org/cgi/content/abstract/134/4/p62004; "This regimen **reduces corticosteroid requirements** in sarcoidosis with little treatment complication."

Menon RT, Feferman T, Aricha R, Souroujon MC, Fuchs S. "Suppression of experimental autoimmune myasthenia gravis by combination therapy: pentoxifylline as a steroid-sparing agent." J Neuroimmunol. 2008 Sep 15;201-202:128-35 [Erratum in: J Neuroimmunol. 2009 Oct 30;215(1-2):129]; "… we evaluated the therapeutic potential of a combination of suboptimal doses of methylprednisolone (Solumedrol) and Pentoxifylline (PTX), a general phosphodiesterase (PDE) inhibitor, in rat experimental autoimmune MG [myasthenia gravis] (EAMG). This combined treatment resulted in a pronounced suppressive effect on EAMG and was by **far more effective than each of the drugs administered separately at these low doses**. … This study demonstrates **the potential of PTX [pentoxifylline] as a steroid-sparing agent** in the management of myasthenia gravis."

Han J, Thompson P, Beutler B. "Dexamethasone and pentoxifylline inhibit endotoxin-induced cachectin/ tumor necrosis factor synthesis at separate points in the signaling pathway." J Exp Med. 1990 Jul 1;172(1):391-4; "… In RAW 264.7 macrophages, **pentoxifylline blocks cachectin/** [tumor necrosis factor] **TNF** [microsomal ribonucleic acid] **mRNA accumulation** but has no effect upon the efficiency of reporter mRNA translation. Dexamethasone, on the other hand, has only a modest effect on cachectin/ TNF mRNA accumulation, but strongly impedes translational derepression. **Combined application of dexamethasone and pentoxifylline to macrophages causes a greater suppression of cachectin/ TNF biosynthesis that can be achieved by either agent**

alone. ..."

The abstracts listed below suggest, specifically, the safety, of pentoxifylline in its many forms.

Smart L, Gobejishvili L, Crittenden N, Barve S, McClain CJ. "Alcoholic Hepatitis: Steroids vs. Pentoxifylline." Curr Hepat Rep. 2013 Mar 1;12(1):59-65; an excellent review of "the mechanisms and rationale for use" of **pentoxifylline**, which is noted as **"a relatively innocuous therapeutic agent" that addresses "multi-system organ failure"**; available free on the web at
http://link.springer.com/article/10.1007/s11901-012-0158-y/fulltext.html

Haque KN, Pammi M "Pentoxifylline for treatment of sepsis and necrotizing enterocolitis in neonates." Cochrane Database Syst Rev. 2011 Oct 5; "... 227 neonates with suspected or confirmed sepsis were randomised to pentoxifylline or placebo. Pentoxifylline therapy significantly decreased 'all cause mortality during hospital stay' in the overall population of infants with sepsis .... Subgroup analyses revealed **significant reduction in mortality in preterm infants, infants with confirmed sepsis and gram-negative sepsis. ... No adverse effects due to pentoxifylline were noted**. ..."

Harris E, Schulzke SM, Patole SK. "Pentoxifylline in preterm neonates: a systematic review." Paediatr Drugs. 2010 Oct 1;12(5):301-11.

MSDS [material safety data sheet]. "Pentoxifylline." ChemWatch#sc-203184; 14-FEB-2009; "animal experiments indicate that ingestion of less than 150 grams may be fatal or may produce serious damage to the health of the individual." [150 grams = 375 of the standard 400 mg ER pentoxifylline tablets].

MSDS [material safety data sheet]. "Pentoxifylline." CAS# [Chemical Abstracts Service number] 6493-05-6; revised 2008; the oral LD_{50} (rat) for pentoxifylline is 1,170 mg/kg, which on the Hodge and Sterner scale would earn it a rating of "slightly toxic".

Erikci AA, Ozturk A, Karagoz B, Bilgi O, Turken O, Top C, Kandemir EG. "Results of combination therapy with amifostine, pentoxifylline, ciprofloxacin and dexamethasone in patients with myelodysplastic syndrome and acute myeloid leukemia." Hematology. 2008 Oct;13(5):289-92 [safely used pentoxifylline **2,400 mg/day**] [the more commonly used dose is 1,200 mg/day]

Incandela L, De Sanctis MT, Cesarone MR, Belcaro G, Nicolaides AN, Geroulakos G, Ramaswami G. "Short-range intermittent claudication and rest pain: microcirculatory effects of pentoxifylline in a randomized, controlled trial." Angiology. 2002 Jan-Feb;53 Suppl 1:S27-30 [safely used pentoxifylline **2,400 mg/day**].

Falanga V, Fujitani RM, Diaz C, Hunter G, Jorizzo J, Lawrence PF, Lee BY, Menzoian JO, Tretbar LL, Holloway GA, Hoballah J, Seabrook GR, McMillan DE, Wolf W. "Systemic treatment of venous leg ulcers with high doses of pentoxifylline: efficacy in a randomized, placebo-controlled trial." Wound Repair Regen. 1999 Jul-Aug;7(4):208-13 [safely used pentoxifylline **2,400 mg/day** – viewed as providing better healing than 1,200 mg/day].

Suárez-Peñaranda JM, Rico-Boquete R, López-Rivadulla M, Blanco-Pampín J, Concheiro-Carro L. "A fatal case of suicidal pentoxifylline intoxication." Int J Legal Med. 1998;111(3):151-3; "It is considered to be a safe drug and to the best of our knowledge there are no reports in the medical literature of cases of fatal poisoning. There is only one previous report of a young woman who tried to commit suicide by taking a large amount of the drug but recovered." [this patient was estimated to have taken about 30,000 mg of pentoxifylline, achieving a blood level about 25 times the norm; the previous report was in Br Med J (Clin Res Ed). 1984 Jan 7;288(6410):26].

The abstracts listed below concern the role of pentoxifylline in regulating the balance of Th1 and Th2 (Thymus-derived lymphocyte helper cells types 1 & 2) – which, for the most part, is not here discussed. While pentoxifylline has been known since

31

at least 1993 to be a selective suppressor of Th1 derived cytokines (interferon gamma, interlukin-2 & tumor necrosis factor beta) and since at least 1995 to be a suppressor at high doses of both Th1 and Th2 derived cytokines (interleukins 4, 5, 9 & 13), the whole question of maintaining – or obtaining – an optimal Th1/ Th2 balance is various autoimmune conditions is still more controversial than one would hope.

Benbernou N, Esnault S, Potron G, Guenounou M. "Regulatory effects of pentoxifylline on T-helper cell-derived cytokine production in human blood cells." J Cardiovasc Pharmacol. 1995;25 Suppl 2:S75-9; "... **PTX [pentoxifylline] at the appropriate concentrations could induce selective suppression of IL-2 [interlukin-2] and IFN-gamma [interferon gamma]**, whereas at high concentrations this drug **[pentoxifylline] could act as a suppressive agent of both Th1- and Th2-derived cytokines**. ..."

Rott O, Cash E, Fleischer B. "**Phosphodiesterase inhibitor pentoxifylline, a selective suppressor of T helper type 1- but not type 2-associated lymphokine production, prevents induction of experimental autoimmune encephalomyelitis** in Lewis rats." Eur J Immunol. 1993 Aug;23(8):1745-51.

RED BLOOD CELL (ANEMIA) & PLATELET (COAGULATION) DISORDERS

The abstracts listed below address the common misconception that pentoxifylline might induce bleeding; actually, pentoxifylline reduces anemia.

Johnson DW, Pascoe EM, Badve SV, Dalziel K, Cass A, Clarke P, Ferrari P, McDonald SP, Morrish AT, Pedagogos E, Perkovic V, Reidlinger D, Scaria A, Walker R, Vergara LA, Hawley CM; HERO Study Collaborative Group. "A Randomized, Placebo-Controlled Trial of Pentoxifylline on Erythropoiesis-Stimulating Agent Hyporesponsiveness in Anemic Patients With CKD [chronic kidney disease]: The Handling Erythropoietin

Resistance With Oxpentifylline (HERO) Trial." Am J Kidney Dis. 2015 Jan;65(1):49-57; "…Pentoxifylline (400 mg/d; n=26) or matching placebo (control; n=27) for 4 months. … **Pentoxifylline significantly increased hemoglobin concentration** relative to the control group … ." [note that the dose used was one-third of the more commonly used dose]

Mohammadpour AH, Nazemian F, Khaiat MH, Tafaghodi M, Salari P, Charkazi S, Naghibi M, Shamsara J. "Evaluation of the effect of pentoxifylline on erythropoietin-resistant anemia in hemodialysis patients." Saudi J Kidney Dis Transpl. 2014 Jan-Feb;25(1):73-8; "…This prospective study to evaluate the effect of pentoxyphylline on erythropoeisis was performed on 15 (eight males, seven females) clinically stable patients who had been on hemodialysis for at least six months with anemia (Hgb of <10.7 g/dL) unresponsive to rh-Epo despite high doses. They were treated with 400 mg pentoxifylline tablets once daily for 12 weeks. **Hgb [hemoglobin] increased after one and two months of drug administration, but significant changes were observed in eight (53%) patients after three months** .…" [note that the dose used was one-third of the most commonly used dose]

Jennings DL, Wlliams CT, Morgan JA. "Pentoxifylline for the treatment of hemolytic anemia in a patient who developed recurrent gastrointestinal bleeding while on continuous-flow left ventricular assist device support." ASAIO J. 2013 Sep-Oct;59(5):526-7; "…a case of a patient with hemolytic anemia after continuous-flow left ventricular assist device (CF-LVAD) implantation that was successfully treated with pentoxifylline. … On October 25, 2011, she was readmitted with anemia and hemoglobin of 6.6 mg/dl and no identifiable source of bleeding. Her lactate dehydrogenase (LDH) was 936 IU/L, indicating severe hemolysis. Due to her evidence of hemolytic anemia and her inability to tolerate antiplatelet therapy due to recurrent bleeding, she was discharged on pentoxifylline 400 mg thrice daily on October 27, 2011, with hemoglobin of 11.2 mg/dl after transfusion. After 60 days of pentoxifylline, her hemoglobin and LDH in clinic were 10.1 mg/dl and 223 IU/L, respectively. … Additional analysis of **pentoxifylline as a therapeutic modality to manage hemolytic anemia** after CF-LVAD implantation may be warranted.

Mora-Gutiérrez JM, Ferrer-Nadal A, García-Fernández N. "Effect of pentoxifylline on anaemia control in haemodialysis patients: retrospective observational case-control study." [Article in English, Spanish] Nefrologia. 2013 Jul 19;33(4):524-531; "... Four patients received PTX due to vascular disease and 14 due to refractory anaemia .... **In HD [hemodialysis] patients, PTX [pentoxifylline] in doses of 800 mg/day improves Hb [hemoglobin] significantly and in the short term (3 months) in HD patients (around 61% response) and allows the required ESA [erythropoiesis-stimulating agent] dose to be reduced in the medium-long term. This effect is sustained over time and treatment is tolerated well.**" [note that the dose used was two-thirds of the more commonly used dose]

Ueno M, Ferreiro JL, Tomasello SD, Tello-Montoliu A, Capodanno D, Seecheran N, Kodali M, Dharmashankar K, Desai B, Charlton RK, Bass TA, Angiolillo DJ. "Impact of pentoxifylline on platelet function profiles in patients with type 2 diabetes mellitus and coronary artery disease on dual antiplatelet therapy with aspirin and clopidogrel." J Am Coll Cardiol, 2011; 57:1920 [earlier draft in JACC Cardiovasc Interv. 2011 Aug;4(8):905-12]; "... This was a prospective, randomized, double-blind, parallel design study conducted in DM [diabetes mellitus] patients with stable coronary artery disease receiving DAPT [dual antiplatelet therapy = aspirin & clopidogrel]. ... **Adjunctive treatment with pentoxifylline is not associated with increased platelet inhibitory effects** in DM patients with coronary artery disease receiving DAPT."

Assem M, Yousri M. "Impact of pentoxifylline and vitamin E on Ribavirin-induced haemolytic anaemia in chronic hepatitis C patients: an Egyptian survey." Int J Hepatol. 2011:530949; "...Selected 200 naïve chronic HCV [hepatitis C virus] patients, were randomized to receive either the standard antiviral therapy (peginterferon α-2b and RBV [ribavirin]) plus pentoxifylline (800 mg) and high-dose vitamin E (1000 iu) daily (combined group) or received standard antiviral therapy plus placebo only (control group). They were followed ... for 6 months post-treatment .... **Pentoxifylline and vitamin E can ameliorate RBV**

[ribavirin]-associated haemolysis; improve compliance and virologic clearance when combined with the standard antiviral therapy in patients with chronic hepatitis C." [note that the dose used was two-thirds of the more commonly used dose] [see also Euroasian J Hepato-Gastroenterol. Jan-Jun 2012;2(1):35-40]

Adel M, Awad HA, Abdel-Naim AB, Al-Azizi MM. "Effects of pentoxifylline on coagulation profile and disseminated intravascular coagulation incidence in Egyptian septic neonates." J Clin Pharm Ther. 2010 Jun;35(3):257-65; "**Pentoxifylline protects against sepsis-induced microcirculatory derangement in neonates. It significantly lowered the incidence of bleeding and MODS [multiple organ dysfunction syndrome] and shortened the length of hospital stay.**"

Golbasi I, Akbas H, Ozdem S, Ukan S, Ozdem SS, Kabukçu H, Turkay C, Bayezid O. "The effect of pentoxifylline on haemolysis during cardiopulmonary bypass in open-heart surgery." Acta Cardiol. 2006 Feb;61(1):7-11; "PTX **[pentoxifylline] may be an effective agent in reducing the haemolysis** during CPB [cardiopulmonary bypass]."

Dart RC, ed. Medical Toxicology. 3rd ed. Philadelphia: Lippincott Williams & Wilkins, 2004; p.633: "Because pentoxifylline reduces blood viscosity and affects platelet aggregation and fibrinogen levels, it might be expected to exacerbate any ongoing bleeding. However, **there have been no reports of significant hemorrhage associated with either overdose or therapeutic use. Therapeutic doses do not appear to significantly affect any of the coagulation parameters, even in patients on concomitant warfarin therapy ....**"

Ingerslev J, Mouritzen C, Stenbjerg S. "**Pentoxifylline does not interfere with stable coumarin anticoagulant therapy**: a clinical study." Pharmatherapeutica. 1986;4(9):595-600.

Iwafune Y, Yoshimoto H. "Clinical use of pentoxifylline in haemorrhagic disorders of the retina." Pharmatherapeutica. 1980;2(7):429-38; "**in the group treated with pentoxifylline, there was significantly earlier** absorption of the haemorrhage ...”; “No side-effects causing haemorrhagic disorders were found.”

KIDNEY (RENAL) DISORDERS (INCLUDING DIABETES MELLITUS)

The abstracts listed below certainly suggest that all those with diabetes mellitus should be on pentoxifylline – but they also suggest that most with a wide variety of renal disorders should be on it – as pentoxifylline reduces the amount of “normal wear and tear” blood cells cause when rushing through an organ's tissues.

Argyropoulos, C. “Pentoxifylline in renal disease, a tour through the literature.” 22 Sep 2014; http://www.pbfluids.com/2014/09/tomorrow-is-another-exciting-edition-of.html ; an astoundingly good review with data charts and 18 references.

Navarro-González JF, Mora-Fernández C, Muros de Fuentes M, Chahin J, Méndez ML, Gallego E, Macía M, Del Castillo N, Rivero A, Getino MA, García P, Jarque A, García J. “Effect of Pentoxifylline on Renal Function and Urinary Albumin Excretion in Patients with Diabetic Kidney Disease: The PREDIAN Trial.” J Am Soc Nephrol. 2015 Jan;26(1):220-9; “... In this population [82 patients, 87 controls], **addition of PTF [pentoxifylline, 1,200 mg/d for 2 years] to RAS [renin-angiotensin system] inhibitors resulted in a smaller decrease in eGFR [estimated glomerular filtration rate] and a greater reduction of residual albuminuria.**”

Chen PM, Lai TS, Chen PY, Lai CF, Wu V, Chiang WC, Chen YM, Wu KD, Tsai TJ. “Renoprotective effect of combining pentoxifylline with angiotensin-converting enzyme inhibitor or angiotensin II receptor blocker in advanced chronic kidney disease.” J Formos Med Assoc. 2014 Feb 7; “... A single-center retrospective analysis .... of 661 Stage 3B-5 CKD patients .... **In the advanced stages of CKD [chronic kidney disease], patients treated with a combination of pentoxifylline and**

ACEI [angiotensin-converting enzyme inhibitor] or ARB [angiotensin II receptor blocker] had a better renal outcome than those treated with ACEI or ARB alone**. This effect was more prominent in the higher proteinuria subgroup. ..."

Nasiri-Toosi Z, Dashti-Khavidaki S, Khalili H, Lessan-Pezeshki M. "A review of the potential protective effects of pentoxifylline against drug-induced nephrotoxicity." Eur J Clin Pharmacol. 2013 May;69(5):1057-73; "... Some possible pharmacologic mechanisms of pentoxifylline (PTX) that suggest it as a candidate to ameliorate AKI [acute kidney injury] include interaction at the level of the adenosine receptors, increase in erythrocyte deformability, stimulation of vasodilatory prostaglandins production and prevention of vascular congestion, and suppression of tumor necrosis factor alpha (TNF-α) and apoptosis. This manuscript **reviews all clinical and animal studies on the use of PTX [pentoxifylline] as a renoprotective agent against a number of nephrotoxic drugs**. ... Although some available animal studies show protective effects of PTX against renal toxicity of some antimicrobial and cytotoxic agents, designing clinical trials to approve these nephroprotective effects requires prior confirmation of no reducing antimicrobial or antitumor action of these medications by PTX."

Badri S, Dashti-Khavidaki S, Ahmadi F, Mahdavi-Mazdeh M, Abbasi MR, Khalili H. "Effect of add-on pentoxifylline on proteinuria in membranous glomerulonephritis: A 6-month placebo-controlled trial." Clin Drug Investig. 2013 Mar;33(3):215-22; "...a double-blind, placebo-controlled trial. ... Non-diabetic patients with histologically proven MGN [membranous glomerulonephritis] and urinary protein excretion (UPE) >500 mg/24 h, entered a 6-month study period. ... **Treatment with pentoxifylline [400 mg 2 or 3 times per day] for 6 months resulted in a significant reduction of mean UPE [urinary protein excretion](p < 0.001) along with a slight, non-significant increase of eGFR [estimated glomerular filtration rate]**, in comparison to the mean UPE and eGFR increase in the placebo group. ..."

Ghorbani A, Omidvar B, Beladi-Mousavi SS, Lak E, Vaziri S. "The effect of pentoxifylline on reduction of proteinuria among patients with type 2 diabetes under blockade of angiotensin system: a double blind and randomized clinical trial." Nefrologia. 2012 Nov 21;32(6):790-796; "… One hundred patients with DN [diabetic nephropathy] and persistent proteinuria despite treatment with losartan and enalapril in at least 3 months before inclusion in the study were randomly assigned to two groups. … In the [400 mg/day] PTX [pentoxifylline] group, the mean rate of urinary protein excretion … significantly decreased from 616.66 mg to 378.24 after 3 months (P=.000) and to 192.05 mg after 6 months (P=.000) whereas no significant changes were observed in the control group. The beneficial antiproteinuric effect of PTX was not associated to the degree of metabolic control and a reduction of blood pressure. … at the end of study, the mean clearance of creatinine was significantly higher in PTX group (P=.04). In conclusion, **PTX [pentoxifylline] can significantly provide additive antiproteinuric effect and slow the decrease in GFR [glomerular filtration rate] among patients with type 2 DM [diabetes mellitus] under blockade of angiotensin system**." [note that the dose used was one-third of the more commonly used dose]

Goicoechea M, García de Vinuesa S, Quiroga B, Verdalles U, Barraca D, Yuste C, Panizo N, Verde E, Muñoz MA, Luño J. "Effects of pentoxifylline on inflammatory parameters in chronic kidney disease patients: a randomized trial." J Nephrol. 2012 Nov;25(6):969-75; "…a prospective randomized trial of 91 patients with estimated glomerular filtration rate (eGFR) <60 ml/min, calculated with 4-variable Modification of Diet in Renal Disease (MDRD-4) Study equation. Patients were randomly assigned to treatment with PTF [pentoxifylline] 400 mg (twice a day) (n=46) or to continue their usual therapy (n=45). Clinical, biochemical and inflammatory parameters were measured at baseline, and at 6 and 12 months of treatment. …. **High-sensitivity C-reactive protein (hs-CRP), serum fibrinogen and TNF-alpha decreased significantly** in patients treated with PTF in comparison with the control group … . Conclusions: **PTF [pentoxifylline] treatment decreases inflammatory markers in chronic kidney disease and stabilizes renal function**." [note that the dose used was two-thirds of the more commonly used dose]

Gonzalez-Espinoza L, Rojas-Campos E, Medina-Pérez M, Peña-Quintero P, Gómez-Navarro B, Cueto-Manzano AM. "Pentoxifylline decreases serum levels of tumor necrosis factor alpha, interleukin 6 and C-reactive protein in hemodialysis patients: results of a randomized double-blind, controlled clinical trial." Nephrol Dial Transplant. (2011) published online 03 October 2011; "...a study (**n** = 18, pentoxifylline 400 mg/day) or control (**n** = 18, placebo) group ... . Pentoxifylline significantly decreased serum concentrations of TNF-α, IL-6 and CRP compared to placebo. **Pentoxifylline could be a promising and useful strategy to reduce the systemic inflammation frequently observed in patients on HD [hemodialysis].**" [note that the dose used was one-third of the more commonly used dose]

Asvadi I, Hajipour B, Asvadi A, Asl NA, Roshangar L, Khodadadi A. "Protective effect of pentoxyfilline in renal toxicity after methotrexate administration." Eur Rev Med Pharmacol Sci. 2011 Sep;15(9):1003-9; "... Forty five male Wistar **rats** were assigned to 3 groups of 15 animals each: Group 1: control group (0.9% saline). Group 2: MTX [methotrexate]; injected with 20 mg/kg MTX intraperitoneally (i.p.). Group 3: MTX + PTX [pentoxifylline] injected i.p. MTX (20 mg/kg) + PTX (50 mg/kg) i.p. PTX was administered since 3 days before MTX administration and continued for 6 days. ... **PTX [pentoxifylline] administration ... attenuated renal tissue injury and number of apoptic cells and suppressed the elevation of BUN [blood urea nitrogen and Cr [creatinine] levels. ...**"

Barkhordari K, Karimi A, Shafiee A, Soltaninia H, Khatami MR, Abbasi K, Yousefshahi F, Haghighat B, Brown V. "Effect of pentoxifylline on preventing acute kidney injury after cardiac surgery by measuring urinary neutrophil gelatinase - associated lipocalin." J Cardiothorac Surg. 2011 Jan 19;6(1):8; "...PTX [pentoxifylline] had a positive effect in preventing AKI [acute kidney injury] reflecting in changes in sCr [serum creatinine] , and the increase of UNGAL [urinary neutrophil gelatinase-associated lipocalin] was consistent with the emergence of AKI ... . **PTX [pentoxifylline] could reduce the occurrence of AKI [acute kidney** injury] as determined by attenuation of sCr [serum creatinine] rise without causing hemodynamic instability or increased bleeding. ..."

Oliaei F1, Hushmand S2, Khafri S3, Baradaran M4. "Efficacy of pentoxifylline for reduction of proteinuria in type II diabetic patients." Caspian J Intern Med. 2011 Fall;2(4):309-13;"... this randomized clinical trial study was performed on 60 type II diabetic patients with proteinuria over 500 mg/day despite receiving angiotensin receptor or angiotensin converting enzyme inhibitors. These patients were randomly divided into group A (Placebo) and group B (Pentoxifylline 400 mg 3 times daily). ... The reduction of proteinuria in placebo group was 294 ± 497 mg/dl and in the case group was 979 ± 695 mg/dl ($p<0.05$). The mean creatinine clearance in placebo group was 79.4 ± 19.9 and in the case group was 80.6 ± 22.8 mL/min .... The results show that **adding pentoxifylline to other approved angiotensin system inhibitors can significantly reduce proteinuria in diabetic nephropathy and influence progression of the disease with no effect on renal function.**"

Badri S, Dashti-Khavidaki S, Lessan-Pezeshki M, Abdollahi M. "A review of the potential benefits of pentoxifylline in diabetic and non-diabetic proteinuria." J Pharm Pharm Sci. 2011;14(1):128-37; "... **Pentoxifylline (PTF) is known for its potent inhibitory effects against cell proliferation and inflammation** which play important roles in CKD [chronic kidney disease] progression. Data derived from both human studies and animal models demonstrated that **PTF has broad-spectrum renoprotective effects** and therefore, provide a scientific basis for the use of PTF as an anti-proteinuric agent. Conclusion of this review is that **short-term use of PTF may produce a significant reduction of proteinuria in subjects with diabetic and also non-diabetic kidney diseases** but the **reports of long-term use of PTF also show that urinary protein excretion exhibits a progressive and sustained reduction in patients treated with PTF. ...**"

Renke M, Tylicki L, Rutkowski P, Knap N, Zietkiewicz M, Neuwelt A, Aleksandrowicz E, Łysiak-Szydłowska W, Woźniak M, Rutkowski B. "Effect of pentoxifylline on proteinuria, markers of tubular injury and oxidative stress in non-diabetic patients with chronic kidney disease - placebo controlled, randomized, cross-over study." Acta Biochim Pol. 2010;57(1):119-23; **"The PTE [pentoxifylline] therapy reduced proteinuria (by 26 %) as compared to placebo."**

Han KH, Han SY, Kim HS, Kang YS, Cha DR. "Prolonged administration enhances the renoprotective effect of pentoxifylline via anti-inflammatory activity in streptozotocin-induced diabetic nephropathy." Inflammation. 2010 Jun;33(3):137-43; "... in diabetic **rats**, administration of PTX [pentoxifylline] for 4 weeks **inhibited the renal inflammatory reaction**, and when administration for 8 weeks, it **prevented proteinuria**. These findings support the hypothesis that **prolonged administration enhances the protective effects of PTX [pentoxifylline]**." [this increasing effect with time has been noted in other studies; the current study is confirming]

Ferrari P, Mallon D, Trinder D, Olynyk JK. "Pentoxifylline improves haemoglobin and interleukin-6 levels in chronic kidney disease." Nephrology (Carlton). 2010 Apr;15(3):344-9; "Pentoxifylline reduces circulating IL-6 and **improves haemoglobin in non-inflammatory moderate to severe CKD [chronic kidney disease]**. These changes are associated with changes in circulating transferrin saturation and ferritin, suggesting improved iron release. It is hypothesized that pentoxifylline improves iron disposition possibly through modulation of hepcidin."

Roozbeh J, Banihashemi MA, Ghezlou M, Afshariani R, Salari S, Moini M, Sagheb MM. "Captopril and combination therapy of captopril and pentoxifylline in reducing proteinuria in diabetic nephropathy." Ren Fail. 2010 Jan;32(2):172-8: **"The difference in reduction [of proteinuria] only started after two months of pentoxifylline use"**; **"Combining an angiotensin-converting enzyme inhibitor and pentoxifylline can lead to a greater reduction in proteinuria."**

Leyva-Jiménez R, Rodríguez-Orozco AR, Ortega-Pierres LE, Ramírez-Enríquez J, Gómez-García A, Alvarez-Aguilar C. ["Effect of pentoxifylline on the evolution of diabetic nephropathy"] [article in Spanish; abstract in English is per www.pubmed.gov]. Med Clin (Barc).

2009 May 30;132(20):772-8; **"PXF [pentoxifylline] should be used in the preventive treatment of DN [diabetic nephropathy].** These results showed that inflammation and pro-inflammatory cytokines are related to the progression of diabetic nephropathy."

Perkins RM, Aboudara MC, Uy AL, Olson SW, Cushner HM, Yuan CM. "Effect of pentoxifylline on GFR decline in CKD: a pilot, double-blind, randomized, placebo-controlled trial." Am J Kidney Dis. 2009 Apr;53(4):606-16; **"For pentoxifylline-treated participants, the mean estimated GFR [glomerular filtration rate] decrease during treatment was slower compared with the year before study enrollment ...."**

Rodríguez-Morán M, Guerrero-Romero F. "Efficacy of pentoxifylline in the management of microalbuminuria in patients with diabetes." Curr Diabetes Rev. 2008 Feb;4(1):55-62; "Pentoxifylline, a xanthine derivate drug with hemorheologic properties ... is also an antagonist of adenosine 2 receptors and has anti-inflammatory and immunomodulatory effects, properties that promote beneficial changes in the blood flow conditions and kidney function"; "pentoxifylline has low side-effects, **reduces both proteinuria and microalbuminuria in subjects with diabetes**, and is as effective as captopril in the reduction of microalbuminuria in non-hypertensive type 2 diabetic patients."

Mettang T, Krumme B, Bohler J, Roeckel A. "Pentoxifylline as treatment for uraemic pruritus – an addition to the weak armentarium for a common clinical symptom?" Nephrol Dial Transplant. 2007 Sep;22(9):2727-8; "...PTX [pentoxifylline] 600 mg (Trental) was administered intravenously using the venous blood line during the last hour of each dialysis session, over a period of 4 weeks. ... The treatment course was completely administered in three patients and in these three, **pruritus was reduced dramatically** ... . While in the first week almost no effect could be noted, **reduction of pruritus started in the second week and reached its peak during the third week. In two patients, the effect continued over at least two more weeks after discontinuation of the treatment**. ..." [note that the dose used was one-half of the more commonly used dose]

Maiti R, Agrawal NK, Dash D, Pandey BL. "Effect of Pentoxifylline on inflammatory burden, oxidative stress and platelet aggregability in hypertensive type 2 diabetes mellitus patients." Vascul Pharmacol. 2007 Aug-Sep;47(2-3):118-24; **"in the Pentoxifylline group, there was 20.9% decrease ... in C-reactive protein, 18% reduction ... in erythrocyte sedimentation rate, 11.1% reduction ... in total leukocyte count and 5.8% increase ... in serum albumin."**

Rodriguez-Morán M, González-González G, Bermúdez-Barba MV, Medina de la Garza CE, Tamez-Pérez HE, Martínez-Martínez FJ, Guerrero-Romero F. "Effects of pentoxifylline on the urinary protein excretion profile of type 2 diabetic patients with microproteinuria: a double-blind, placebo-controlled randomized trial." Clin Nephrol. 2006 Jul;66(1):3-10; **"Pentoxifylline reduces the excretion of both high and low molecular-weight urinary proteins."**

Lin SL, Chiang WC, Chen YM, Lai CF, Tsai TJ, Hsieh BS. "The renoprotective potential of pentoxifylline in chronic kidney disease." J Chin Med Assoc. 2005 Mar;68(3):99-105; http://homepage.vghtpe.gov.tw/~jcma/68/3/99.pdf; p.105, figure 1: "The renoprotective mechanisms of pentoxifylline in the treatment of chronic kidney disease" – **an excellent schematic overview of the 6 areas in renal pathophysiology where pentoxifylline has demonstrated action**:

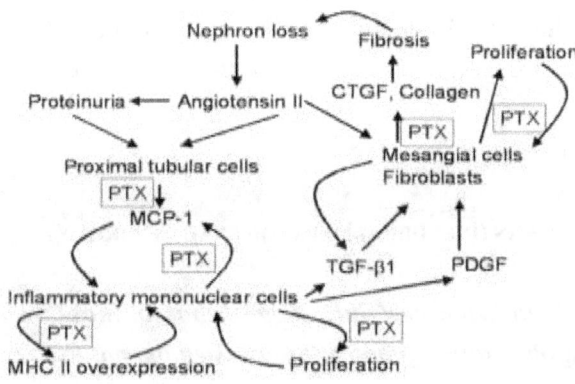

"Pentoxifylline, a non-selective phosphodiesterase inhibitor with indiscernible toxicity, exerts potent inhibitory effects against cell

43

proliferation, inflammation, and extracellular matrix accumulation, all of which play important roles in CKD progression. **Pentoxifylline monotherapy markedly reduces proteinuria in patients with membranous nephropathy.** Moreover, **limited human studies have proven pentoxifylline efficacy in reducing proteinuria in patients with diabetes receiving angiotensin-converting enzyme inhibitors, and in patients with nephrotic syndrome secondary to lupus nephritis** despite immunosuppressive therapy."

Navarro JF, Mora C, Muros M, García J. "Additive antiproteinuric effect of pentoxifylline in patients with type 2 diabetes under angiotensin II receptor blockade: a short-term, randomized, controlled trial." J Am Soc Nephrol. 2005 Jul;16(7):2119-26;, "administration of PTF [pentoxifylline] to patients who have type 2 diabetes and are under long-term treatment with an ARB [angiotensin receptor blocker] produces **a significant additive antiproteinuric effect** associated with a reduction of urinary TNF-alpha excretion."

Galindo-Rodríguez G, Bustamante R, Esquivel-Nava G, Salazar-Exaire D, Vela-Ojeda J, Vadillo-Buenfil M, Aviña-Zubieta JA. "Pentoxifylline in the treatment of refractory nephrotic syndrome secondary to lupus nephritis." J Rheumatol. 2003 Nov;30(11):2382-4; "...All [11] patients had received corticosteroids and immunosuppressants for at least 6 months. **All patients showed a decrease in proteinuria concentrations after use of pentoxifylline** [800-1,600 mg/d] from a median of 5.5 to 2.0 ...." [note that the dose used was two-thirds to four-thirds of the more commonly used dose]

LIVER (HEPATIC) DISORDERS (INCLUDING HEPATORENAL SYNDROME)

The abstracts listed below certainly suggest that all those with alcoholic steatohepatitis, nonalcoholic steatohepatitis, or hepatorenal syndrome should be on pentoxifylline – but they also suggest that most with a wide variety of hepatic disorders should be on it – as pentoxifylline reduces the amount of

44

"normal wear and tear" blood cells cause when rushing through an organ's tissues.

Mathurin P, Louvet A, Duhamel A, Nahon P, Carbonell N, Boursier J, Anty R, Diaz E, Thabut D, Moirand R, Lebrec D, Moreno C, Talbodec N, Paupard T, Naveau S, Silvain C, Pageaux GP, Sobesky R, Canva-Delcambre V, Dharancy S, Salleron J, Dao T. "Prednisolone with vs without pentoxifylline and survival of patients with severe alcoholic hepatitis: a randomized clinical trial." JAMA. 2013 Sep 11;310(10):1033-41: "...[270] Patients were randomly assigned to receive either a combination of 40 mg of prednisolone once a day and 400 mg of pentoxifylline 3 times a day (n=133) for 28 days, or 40 mg of prednisolone and matching placebo (n=137) for 28 days. ... The study may have been underpowered to detect a significant difference in incidence of **hepatorenal syndrome, which was less frequent in the group receiving pentoxifylline."**

Zein CO, Lopez R, Kirwan JP, Yerian LM, McCullough AJ, Hazen SL, Feldstein AE. "Pentoxifylline decreases oxidized lipid products in nonalcoholic steatohepatitis: New evidence on the potential therapeutic mechanism." Hepatology. 2012 Oct;56(4):1291-9; "... PTX [pentoxifylline] is known to decrease free-radical mediated oxidative stress and inhibit lipid oxidation. ... Therapy with PTX resulted in significant decreases on 9-HODE [9-hydroxyoctadecadenoic acid] and 13-oxoODE [13-octadecadienoic acid], oxidized lipid products of linoleic acid (LA) linked to histological severity in NAFLD [**Non-alcoholic fatty liver disease**]. Similarly, PTX therapy was associated with significant decreases in 8-HETE [8-hydroxyeicosatetraenoic acid], 9-HETE, and 11-HETE compared to placebo. **Statistically significant correlations were demonstrated between the decrease in HODEs and oxoODEs [oxidized lipid products] and improved histological scores of [hepatic] fibrosis; and between the decrease in HETEs [other oxidized lipid products] and improved [hepatic] lobular inflammation. ..."**

Kianifar HR, Khalesi M, Mahmoodi E, Afzal Aghaei M. "Pentoxifylline in hepatopulmonary syndrome." World J Gastroenterol. 2012 Sep

21;18(35):4912-6; "... 10 **children with chronic liver disease, who had HPS [hepatopulmonary syndrome]**, 20 mg/kg/d PTX [pentoxifylline] was administered for 3 mo. . **Among patients who could tolerate PTX [6 of the 10], there was a significant increase in arterial oxygen pressure (PaO(2)) ... and oxygen saturation (SaO(2)) ... and alveolar-arterial oxygen gradient** ... after 3 mo of treatment. Significant decreases in PaO(2) ... and alveolar-arterial oxygen gradient ... were also seen after drug discontinuation. ... "

Li W, Zheng L, Sheng C, Cheng X, Qing L, Qu S. "Systematic review on the treatment of pentoxifylline in patients with non-alcoholic fatty liver disease." Lipids Health Dis. 2011 Apr 8;10(1):49.; "... **Pentoxifylline - treated patients showed a significant decrease in AST ... and ALT [enzymes whose elevation suggests liver disease] ... ."**

Zein CO, Yerian LM, Gogate P, Lopez R, Kirwan J, Feldstein AE, McCullough AJ. "Pentoxifylline improves nonalcoholic steatohepatitis: A randomized placebo-controlled trial." Hepatology. 2011 Jul 11; "... 55 **adults with biopsy-confirmed NASH** were randomized to receive PTX [pentoxifylline] at a dose of 400 mg three times a day (n=26) or placebo (n=29) over 1 year. ... **PTX [pentoxifylline] significantly improved steatosis ... and lobular inflammation ... . PTX also improved liver fibrosis ... ."**

Tyagi P, Sharma P, Sharma BC, Puri AS, Kumar A, Sarin SK. "Prevention of hepatorenal syndrome in patients with cirrhosis and ascites: a pilot randomized control trial between pentoxifylline and placebo." Eur J Gastroenterol Hepatol. 2011 Mar;23(3):210-7; "... [randomized controlled; 61 of 70 patients completed the 6-month study] **Pentoxifylline is effective in preventing HRS [hepatorenal syndrome] in patients with cirrhosis and ascites at risk of HRS."**

Frazier TH, Stocker AM, Kershner NA, Marsano LS, McClain CJ. "Treatment of alcoholic liver disease." Therap Adv Gastroenterol. 2011 Jan;4(1):63-81; "... **Pentoxifylline appears to be especially effective in ALD [alcoholic liver disease] patients with renal dysfunction/**

hepatorenal syndrome. Biologics such as specific anti-TNFs have been disappointing and should probably not be used outside of the clinical trial setting. ... ".

Petrowsky H, Breitenstein S, Slankamenac K, Vetter D, Lehmann K, Heinrich S, DeOliveira ML, Jochum W, Weishaupt D, Frauenfelder T, Graf R, Clavien PA. "Effects of pentoxifylline on liver regeneration: a double-blinded, randomized, controlled trial in 101 patients undergoing major liver resection." Ann Surg. 2010 Nov;252(5):813-22; "Recent experimental data suggest that PTX [pentoxifylline], a tumor necrosis factor (TNF) α inhibitor, **enhances liver regeneration and reduces ischemic injury** through activation of the interleukin-6 (IL-6) signaling pathway. ... One hundred one consecutive noncirrhotic patients undergoing major liver surgery with inflow occlusion were included in a double-blinded, randomized, controlled trial (RCT) at a single tertiary care center (2006-2009). ... Postoperative alanine aminotransferase (AST) levels were significantly decreased for the PTX group on the second postoperative day ... . The study demonstrates **beneficial effects of PTX [pentoxifylline] on regeneration of small remnant livers** ... that seems to be mediated by IL-6."

Kendrick SF, Day CP. "Liver: Can pentoxifylline secure its place in liver therapeutics?" Nat Rev Gastroenterol Hepatol. 2010 Nov;7(11):593-4; "...Results published by the Pentocir study group suggest that pentoxifylline may have found its role" [reference is to Lebrec D, Thabut D, Oberti F, Perarnau JM, Condat B, Barraud H, Saliba F, Carbonell N, Renard P, Ramond MJ, Moreau R, Poynard T; Pentocir Group. **"Pentoxifylline does not decrease short-term mortality but does reduce complications in patients with advanced cirrhosis."** Gastroenterology. 2010 May;138(5):1755-62].

Amini M, Runyon BA. "Alcoholic hepatitis 2010: A clinician's guide to diagnosis and therapy." World J Gastroenterol. 2010 Oct 21;16(39):4905-12; "the efficacy of pentoxifylline has become increasingly apparent"; **"We conclude that the routine use of glucocorticoids for severe AH [alcoholic hepatitis] poses significant risk with equivocal benefit, and**

that pentoxifylline is a better, safer, and cheaper alternative."

Vician M, Olejník J, Gergel M, Brychta I, Michalka P, Jakubovský J. ["Changes in membrane enzymes in warm liver ischemia"]. [article in Czech; abstract in English is per www.pubmed.gov] Rozhl Chir. 2010 Oct;89(10):647-53; "...intravenous administration of **Pentoxifylline and Stobadine [an antioxidant] probably protects the [pig] liver from warm ischemia injury.**" [this is an on-going set of studies in liver transplantation] [research on stobadine and pentoxifylline are proceeding somewhat in tandem as both impact nitric oxide production]

Zein CO. "Pentoxifyline improves non-alcoholic steatohepatitis: Results of a double-blinded, randomized, placebo-controlled trial." Am J Gastroenterol 2010;105[suppl 1]:S114. Abstract 308

Mihaila RG, Nedelcu L, Fratila O, Rezi EC, Domnariu C, Deac M. "Effects of lovastatin and pentoxyphyllin [sic] in nonalcoholic steatohepatitis." Hepatogastroenterology. 2009 Jul-Aug;56(93):1117-21; **"In the pentoxyphyllin-treated group, transaminases [liver enzymes] significantly decreased after 1 month.**"

De BK, Gangopadhyay S, Dutta D, Baksi SD, Pani A, Ghosh P. "Pentoxifylline versus prednisolone for severe alcoholic hepatitis: a randomized controlled trial." World J Gastroenterol. 2009 Apr 7;15(13):1613-9; **"Reduced mortality, improved risk-benefit profile and renoprotective effects of pentoxifylline compared with prednisolone suggest that pentoxifylline is superior to prednisolone for treatment of severe alcoholic hepatitis.**"

Akriviadis E, Botla R, Briggs W, Han S, Reynolds T, Shakil O. "Pentoxifylline improves short-term survival in severe acute alcoholic hepatitis: a double-blind, placebo-controlled trial." Gastroenterology. 2000 Dec;119(6):1637-48; "... **Treatment with PTX [pentoxifylline] improves short-term survival in patients with severe alcoholic hepatitis. The benefit appears to be related to a significant decrease in the risk of developing hepatorenal syndrome. Increasing TNF levels** during the hospital course are associated with an increase in mortality rate." [according to Google Scholar, accessed on 11-FEB-11, **this is the article on pentoxifylline, other than a 1987 review, most cited overall and per year**] [the following abstract of an editorial comment is clearer than the original article's abstract:] Karnam US, Reddy KR. "A toast to pentoxifylline." Am J Gastroenterol. 2001 May;96(5):1635-7; "The aim of this study was to evaluate the efficacy of pentoxifylline in patients with severe acute alcoholic hepatitis. **Pentoxifylline is a nonselective phosphodiesterase inhibitor that decreases tumor necrosis factor (TNF) gene transcription.** ... The study was a prospective, double blind, randomized, placebo-controlled study. The two primary endpoints were the effect of pentoxifylline on 1) the short term survival (during the index hospitalization or over the 28-day study period) and 2) progression to hepatorenal syndrome (HRS). ... **One hundred two patients were enrolled and randomized** to receive either pentoxifylline 400 mg t.i.d. for 4 wk or a placebo. ... In this study, **25% and 46% in the pentoxifylline and control arms died ... . In the patients who died, hepatic failure with HRS [hepatorenal syndrome] had developed in 50% in the pentoxifylline group and 92% in the control group. New onset renal failure occurred in 11% and 43% in the pentoxifylline and control groups, respectively ... and progressed to HRS in 80% and 90% of patients, respectively, in the two groups ...**"

Vázquez García MJ, Vargas Camaño ME, Olalde Carmona R. ["Use of pentoxifylline in pediatric patients with grade IV (OMS) lupus nephropathy who have received multiple treatments"] [article in Spanish; abstract in English is per www.pubmed.gov]. Rev Alerg Mex. 2000 May-Jun;47(3):109-14.

McHutchison JG, Runyon BA, Draguesku JO, Cominelli F, Person JL, Castracane J. "Pentoxifylline may prevent renal impairment (hepatorenal syndrome) in severe acute alcoholic hepatitis." [abstract of presentation at the American Association for the Study of Liver Diseases] Hepatology. 1991;14:96A; "... randomized pilot study, 22 patients with severe AH [alcoholic hepatitis] ... received pentoxifylline ["(1,200 mg po daily) for 10 days"] (which inhibits TNF and interleukins in vitro) or standard

49

treatment. … **The pentoxifylline group developed significantly less renal impairment and fever. … Thirty day mortality was higher in controls compared to treated patients** (1 vs 3, p=NS). …" [this appears to be the study that started this entire line of inquiry, which then was encouraged by a study in mice: Shirin H, Bruck R, Aeed H, Frenkel D, Kenet G, Zaidel L, Avni Y, Halpern Z, Hershkoviz R. "Pentoxifylline prevents concanavalin A-induced hepatitis by reducing tumor necrosis factor alpha levels and inhibiting adhesion of T lymphocytes to extracellular matrix." J Hepatol 1998;29(1):60-7.]

PANCREATIC & INTESTINAL DISORDERS

The abstracts listed below are few but significant; pancreatic and intestinal disorders can be notably hard to treat successfully.

Mostafa TM, Ibrahim OM, Badra GA, Abdallah MS. "Role of pentoxifylline and sparfloxacin in prophylaxis of spontaneous bacterial peritonitis in cirrhotic patients." ISRN Gastroenterol. 2014 Mar 6;2014:595213; "… Forty cirrhotic patients with ascites were included in the study. Patients were randomized into four groups in a blind fashion; each group consists of ten patients. Group one received ciprofloxacin (control group), group two received sparfloxacin, group three received pentoxifylline, and group four received a combination of sparfloxacin and pentoxifylline. Treatment duration was six months. … The finding from our study indicates that sparfloxacin as well as **pentoxifylline could be used in prophylaxis of spontaneous bacterial peritonitis.** Combination of sparfloxacin and pentoxifylline showed some of synergism **which may be useful in decreasing emergence of resistant strains.**"

Le Campion ER, Jukemura J, Coelho AM, Patzina R, Carneiro D'Albuquerque LA. "Effects of intravenous administration of pentoxifylline in pancreatic ischaemia-reperfusion injury." HPB (Oxford). 2013 Aug;15(8):588-94; "… a **rat** model … . **Pentoxifylline administration reduced the systemic inflammatory response, the pancreatic histological lesion and renal dysfunction in pancreatic I-R** [ischaemia-reperfusion] injury and may be a useful tool in pancreas and kidney transplantation."

Lloris Carsi JM, Cejalvo Lapeña D, Toledo AH, Zaragoza Fernandez C, Toledo Pereyra LH. "Pentoxifylline protects the **small intestine** after **severe ischemia and reperfusion**." Exp Clin Transplant. 2013 Jun;11(3):250-8; "… a **rat** model … . **Survival was significantly better at 7 days (70% vs 40%)** when we compared the pentoxifylline group treated at reperfusion (10 mg/kg) to the ischemic controls. …"

Escobar J, Pereda J, Arduini A, Sandoval J, Moreno ML, Pérez S, Sabater L, Aparisi L, Cassinello N, Hidalgo J, Joosten LA, Vento M, López-Rodas G, Sastre J. "Oxidative and nitrosative stress in acute pancreatitis modulation by pentoxifylline and oxypurinol." Biochem Pharmacol. 2011 Oct 8; "… We report here that **oxidative stress and nitrosative stress occur in pancreas and lung in acute pancreatitis and the co-treatment with oxypurinol and pentoxifylline prevents oxidative stress in both tissues**. Oxypurinol was effective in preventing glutathione oxidation, whereas **pentoxyfilline abrogated glutathione depletion**. This latter effect was **independent of TNF-α since glutathione depletion** occurred in **mice** deficient in TNF-α or its receptors after induction of pancreatitis. …"

Peterson TC, Peterson MR, Raoul JM. "The effect of pentoxifylline and its metabolite-1 [hydroxypentoxifylline] on inflammation and fibrosis in the TNBS model of colitis." Eur J Pharmacol. 2011 May 1; "…. The aim of this study was to determine the effect of pentoxifylline and its primary metabolite (M-1) on fibrosis in the TNBS [trinitrobenzene sulfonic acid]-induced colitis model. … Results suggest that **pentoxifylline and M-1 [a metabolite of pentoxifylline] inhibit intestinal fibrosis** in this experimental model and **may prove beneficial in the treatment of intestinal fibrosis associated with human Crohn's disease with the added benefit of inhibiting inflammation and ulceration**. This is the first study to examine the effects of racemic M-1 in vivo and one of the few studies to examine the effect of drugs on both inflammation and fibrosis in an experimental model of colitis."

Sireesh I, Kaman L, Singh R. "Pentoxifylline as an adjuvant to surgery and antibiotics in **the treatment of perforation peritonitis**: a prospective, randomised placebo-controlled study." Singapore Med J. 2008 Aug;49(8):619-23: **"Pentoxifylline improved the outcome by significantly decreasing the length of the hospital stay and the rate of wound infection**."

Lu CH, Chao PC, Borel CO, Yang CP, Yeh CC, Wong CS, Wu CT. "Preincisional intravenous pentoxifylline attenuating perioperative cytokine response, reducing morphine consumption, and improving recovery of bowel function in patients undergoing colorectal cancer surgery." Anesth Analg. 2004 Nov;99(5):1465-71; **"Patients in the PTX [pentoxifylline] group exhibited longer PCA [patient controlled analgesia] trigger times, less morphine consumption, and a faster return of bowel function** compared with patients in the control group."

Murthy S, Cooper HS, Yoshitake H, Meyer C, Meyer CJ, Murthy NS. "Combination therapy of pentoxifylline and TNF-alpha monoclonal antibody in dextran sulphate-induced mouse colitis." Aliment Pharmacol Ther. 1999 Feb;13(2):251-60; "... **The simultaneous administration of pentoxifylline and TNF-alpha mab [monoclonal antibody; (25 microg/mouse, Endogen)] may enhance therapeutic outcomes in inflammatory bowel disease and reduce the side-effects associated with the repeated use of TNF-alpha mab**."

HEART (CARDIAC) DISORDERS

The abstracts listed below suggest that those with congestive heart failure or coronary artery disease – and a variety of other cardiac disorders – might benefit from being placed on pentoxifylline.

Champion S, Lapidus N, Cherié G, Spagnoli V, Oliary J, Solal AC. "Pentoxifylline in heart failure: a meta-analysis of clinical trials."

Cardiovasc Ther. 2014 Aug;32(4):159-62; "… Data from a total of 221 patients with LVEF [left ventricular ejection fraction] ≤40% from six randomized controlled trials were included in this analysis. Pentoxifylline 1,200 mg per day was administered during 6 months, except in one study (administered during 1 month for severe acute HF [heart failure]). … The pooled data including 221 **patients showed a nearly fourfold reduction in mortality [from chronic & acute heart failure] … .**"

Mohammadpour AH, Falsoleiman H, Shamsara J, Allah Abadi G, Rasooli R, Ramezani M. "Pentoxifylline decreases serum level of adhesion molecules in atherosclerosis patients." Iran Biomed J. 2014 Jan;18(1):23-7; "…Clinical studies have indicated that **the level of … adhesion molecules correlates with the severity of atherosclerosis and can predict future cardiovascular events**. … Forty patients with angiographically documented CAD [coronary artery disease], who fulfilled inclusion and exclusion criteria, were entered in the double-blind, randomized, pilot clinical study. … **administration of PTX [pentoxifylline 400 mg tid for 2 months] in CAD [coronary artery disease] patients significantly decreases adhesion molecules [ICAM-1 (intercellular adhesion Molecule 1) & VCAM-1 (vascular cell adhesion molecule 1)] levels.**"

Green LA, Kim C, Gupta SK, Rajashekhar G, Rehman J, Clauss M. "Pentoxifylline reduces TNF-α and HIV-induced vascular endothelial activation." AIDS Res Hum Retroviruses. 2012 Oct;28(10):1207-15; "…in cultivated human lung microvascular endothelial cells. … we found that TNF-α induced VCAM-1 [vascular cell adhesion molecule 1] was reduced **with concentrations of pentoxifylline in the low nanomolar range**, comparable to plasma levels in pentoxifylline treated groups. … **the anti-inflammatory agent pentoxifylline can directly reduce HIV associated pro-inflammatory endothelial activation, which may underlie vascular dysfunction and coronary vascular diseases.**"

Muldowney JA 3rd, Chen Q, Blakemore DL, Vaughan DE. "Pentoxifylline lowers plasminogen activator inhibitor 1 levels in obese individuals: A pilot study." Angiology. 2012 Aug;63(6):429-34;

"**Plasminogen activator inhibitor 1 (PAI-1),** the primary inhibitor of fibrinolysis and C-reactive protein (CRP), **is a predictor of myocardial infarction.** ...Twenty participants were **treated with pentoxifylline .... Plasminogen activator inhibitor 1 ... decreased over the 8-week period** of the study. ..."

Shamsara J, Mohammadpour AH, Behravan J, Falsoleiman H, Ramezani M. "Pentoxifylline decreases soluble CD40 ligand concentration and CD40 gene expression in coronary artery disease patients." Immunopharmacol Immunotoxicol. 2012 Jun;34(3):523-9; "... we evaluated the effect of **2 months pentoxifylline administration in patients with CAD [coronary artery disease].** ... A randomized placebo-controlled double-blind study design was used. Forty CAD patients (32 males and 8 females) were randomized into either 2 months of pentoxifylline treatment (1,200 mg/day) (n = 20) or placebo treatment (n = 20). ... **Pentoxifylline treatment can suppress the CD40/ CD40 ligand system activation** in CAD patients. **As this system has a role in plaque progression and plaque rupture, pentoxifylline could be a good choice for future studies in preventing cardiovascular events.**"

Shamsara J, Behravan J, Falsoleiman H, Mohammadpour AH, Rendeirs J, Ramezani M. "Pentoxifylline administration changes protein expression profile of coronary artery disease patients." Gene. 2011 Nov 1;487(1):107-11; "... Fourteen CAD [coronary artery disease] patients were randomized to 2 months of pentoxifyline treatment (1,200 mg/day) (n=7) or placebo treatment (n=7). Blood samples were obtained before and after treatment. A comparative 2 dimensional gel electrophoresis was performed .... **As the blood mononuclear cell proteome responds to pentoxifylline with changes in a number of atherosclerosis-relevant proteins, it seems that pentoxifylline could be a good choice for future studies for prevention of cardiovascular events.**"

Groesdonk HV, Heringlake M, Heinze H. ["Anti-inflammatory effects of pentoxifylline: importance in cardiac surgery"] [article in German; abstract in English is per www.pubmed.gov]. Anaesthesist. 2009 Nov;58(11):1136-43; "the **perioperative application of this drug** [pentoxifylline] may improve postoperative function of organs at risk, such as the kidneys and liver."

Iskesen I, Kurdal AT, Kahraman N, Cerrahoglu M, Sirin BH. "Preoperative oral pentoxifylline for management of cytokine reactions in cardiac surgery." Heart Surg Forum. 2009 Apr;12(2):E100-4; "[pentoxifylline] has some beneficial effects in protecting the myocardium during the cardioplegic arrest period in open-heart surgery, without affecting postoperative hemodynamics."

Shaw SM, Shah MK, Williams SG, Fildes JE. "Immunological mechanisms of pentoxifylline in chronic heart failure." Eur J Heart Fail. 2009 Feb;11(2):113-8; available free on the web at http://www.ncbi.nlm.nih.gov/pubmed/19168508 "... to date, there have been no clear beneficial effects from TNF-alpha inhibition and indeed trials of direct anti-TNF therapy have provoked worsening of clinical outcomes. Conversely, a possible exception is pentoxifylline (PTX), a putative TNF-alpha inhibitor with possible (but ill-defined) vasodilatory properties. Several small clinical trials assessing the use of PTX [pentoxifylline] in CHF [congestive heart failure] have suggested beneficial effects on multiple surrogate clinical markers. Interestingly, these trials failed to show a concordant effect on circulating TNF despite the clinical improvement, suggesting other key beneficial properties of this novel agent. ..."

Kang YM, Zhang ZH, Xue B, Weiss RM, Felder RB. "Inhibition of brain proinflammatory cytokine synthesis reduces hypothalamic excitation in rats with ischemia-induced heart failure." Am J Physiol Heart Circ Physiol. 2008 Jul;295(1):H227-36; "the finding that **centrally administered pentoxifylline lowers brain proinflammatory cytokines** expands current understanding of cytokine physiology"; "The present study demonstrates conclusively that **a large fraction of the TNF-α and IL-1β that appears in the brains of rats with HF [heart failure] is actually produced inside the blood-brain barrier; brain levels were substantially reduced in pentoxifylline-treated HF rats, but circulating levels were unaffected.**"

Kalantar-Zadeh K, Anker SD, Horwich TB, Fonarow GC. "Nutritional and anti-inflammatory interventions in chronic heart failure." Am J Cardiol. 2008 Jun 2;101(11A):89E-103E; "... Diminished appetite or anorexia and nutritional deficiencies may be both a cause and a consequence of this so-called malnutrition-inflammation-cachexia (MIC) or **wasting syndrome in CHF [congestive heart failure]**. ... Regardless of the etiology of anorexia, **appetite-stimulating agents, especially those with anti-inflammatory properties such as megesterol acetate or pentoxyphylline, may be appropriate adjuncts** to dietary supplementation. ..."

Otani S, Kuinose M, Murakami T, Saito S, Iwagaki H, Tanaka N, Tanemoto K. "Preoperative oral administration of pentoxifylline ameliorates respiratory index after cardiopulmonary bypass through decreased production of IL-6." Acta Med Okayama. 2008 Apr;62(2):69-74: "preoperative daily administration of 900 mg/day **PTX [pentoxifylline]** contributed to the attenuation of CPB [cardiopulmonary bypass]-induced SIRS [systemic inflammatory response syndrome] and **had a beneficial effect on the postoperative course after cardiovascular surgery.**"

Fernandes JL, de Oliveira RT, Mamoni RL, Coelho OR, Nicolau JC, Blotta MH, Serrano CV Jr." Pentoxifylline reduces pro-inflammatory and increases anti-inflammatory activity in **patients with coronary artery disease** – a randomized placebo-controlled study." Atherosclerosis. 2008 Jan;196(1):434-42: "**Pentoxifylline ... significantly reduced the adjusted levels of CRP [C-reactive protein] and TNF-α compared to placebo** after 6 months"; "IL-12 increase was significantly less pronounced with pentoxifylline"; "The levels of the anti-inflammatory cytokine, IL-10, also declined significantly less in the pentoxifylline group compared to placebo"; "**Pentoxifylline reduces pro-inflammatory and increases anti-inflammatory response in patients with ACS [acute coronary syndromes]**".

Heinze H, Rosemann C, Weber C, Heinrichs G, Bahlmann L, Misfeld M,

Heringlake M, Eichler W. "**A single prophylactic dose** of pentoxifylline reduces high dependency unit time in **cardiac surgery** - a prospective randomized and controlled study." Eur J Cardiothorac Surg. 2007 Jul;32(1):83-9; "**Patients treated with PTX [pentoxifylline] could be transferred to a peripheral ward about 24 h earlier than control patients.**"

Zhang M, Xu YJ, Mengi SA, Arneja AS, Dhalla NS. "Therapeutic potentials of pentoxifylline for treatment of cardiovascular diseases." Exp Clin Cardiol. 2004 Summer;9(2):103-11; available free on the web at http://www.ncbi.nlm.nih.gov/pmc/articles/PMC2716262;   "**...PTXF [pentoxifylline] may be used to treat ischemic heart disease because it can improve RBC [red blood cell] deformability, decrease RBC aggregation ..., increase blood flow to the heart ..., and inhibit neutrophil adhesion and the production of some cytokines, such as TNF-α and IL-1 ....** This drug **is also capable of decreasing PAF [platelet-activating factor] levels, reducing the effect of PAF during ischemia-reperfusion injury ..., depressing the proliferation of the VSMC [vascular smooth muscle cells]..., inhibiting platelet aggregation and improving blood flow** .... All these properties of PTXF are interrelated and originate from the inhibition of cAMP PDE [cyclic adenosine monophosphate phosphodiesterase] ....

Sliwa K, Woodiwiss A, Kone VN, Candy G, Badenhorst D, Norton G, Zambakides C, Peters F, Essop R. "Therapy of ischemic cardiomyopathy with the immunomodulating agent pentoxifylline: results of a randomized study." Circulation. 2004 Feb 17;109(6):750-5; "... a single-center, prospective, randomized, double-blind, placebo-controlled study, 38 **patients with ischemic cardiomyopathy** received pentoxifylline 400 mg TID or placebo in addition to standard therapy. Clinical assessment, radionuclide ventriculography, echocardiography, and blood analyses were performed at baseline and after 6 months. ... **Pentoxifylline treatment resulted in an improvement in functional class** (P<0.005) **and an increase in systolic blood pressure** (P<0.005) **and left ventricular radionuclide ejection fraction** (P<0.005) compared with the placebo-treated group. There were **reductions in plasma concentrations** of **CRP [C-reactive protein], NT-pro BNP [N-terminal of the prohormone brain natriuretic peptide], TNF-alpha, and Fas/ Apo-1** in the pentoxifylline compared with the placebo-treated group. ... '

[The extensive and expanding veterinary literature was not thoroughly reviewed, although **one cannot ignore the frequent references to the antiarrhythmic activity of the pentoxifylline structural analogue "propentofylline".**]

Fiedler VB, Komarek JV. "Effects of 1-(5'-oxohexyl)-3-methyl-7-propylxanthine (HWA 285) on viability of ischemic jeopardized myocardium after acute coronary artery occlusion and reperfusion." Arch Int Pharmacodyn Ther. 1981 Nov;254(1):70-84; "...in anesthetized, open-chest dogs in acute experiments. ...**the agent prevented severe arrhythmias during vessel occlusion and reperfusion.** Infarct size and the amount of hemorrhage after flow release both were significantly smaller in the [propentofylline] HWA 285-treated hearts than in saline-treated control hearts (p less than 0.05 in both cases), and the survival rate was higher in the compound group than in the saline controls. These data suggest **a cardioprotective effect** of HWA 285 **in acute canine experiments undergoing coronary artery occlusion and reperfusion, probably due to antiarrhythmic and/ or metabolic properties of the compound. ...**"

LUNG (PULMONARY) DISORDERS

The abstracts listed below emphasize the anti-inflammatory and anti-fibrotic actions of pentoxifylline on lung tissue.

Sunil VR, Vayas KN, Cervelli JA, Malaviya R, Hall L, Massa CB, Gow AJ, Laskin JD, Laskin DL. "Pentoxifylline attenuates nitrogen mustard-induced acute lung injury, oxidative stress and inflammation [**rats**]." Exp Mol Pathol. 2014 Aug;97(1):89-98; "... These data suggest that **pentoxifylline may be useful in treating acute lung injury, inflammation and oxidative stress induced by vesicants.**"

Naranjo TW, Lopera DE, Diaz-Granados LR, Duque JJ, Restrepo M A, Cano LE. "Combined itraconazole-pentoxifylline treatment promptly reduces lung fibrosis induced by chronic pulmonary paracoccidioidomycosis in **mice**." Pulm Pharmacol Ther. 2011 Feb;24(1):81-91; "... In Latin America, chronic pulmonary paracoccidioidomycosis (PCM) is one of the most important, prevalent and systemic fungal diseases that allows the development of lung fibrosis, with the additional disadvantage that this sequel may appear even after an apparently successful course of antifungal therapy. In this study, was propose the pentoxifylline as complementary treatment in the pulmonary PCM due to its immunomodulatory and anti-fibrotic properties demonstrated in vitro and in vivo in liver, skin and lung. ... **When pulmonary paracoccidioidomycosis [a fungal disease] had evolved and reached an advanced stage of disease before treatment began (as normally occurs in many human patients when first diagnosed), the combined therapy (itraconazole plus pentoxifylline) resulted in a significantly more rapid reduction of granulomatous inflammation and pulmonary fibrosis**, when compared with the results of classical antifungal therapy using itraconazole alone."

Zhang XD, Hou JF, Qin XJ, Li WL, Chen HL, Liu R, Liang X, Hai CX. "Pentoxifylline inhibits intercellular adhesion molecule-1 (ICAM-1) and lung injury in experimental phosgene-exposure **rats**." Inhal Toxicol. 2010 Sep;22(11):889-95; "...**PTX [pentoxifylline] reduced phosgene-induced lung injury**, possibly by inhibiting ICAM-1 differential expression."

Shukla D, Chakraborty S, Singh S, Mishra B. "**Doxofylline [the M-5 metabolite of pentoxifylline]**: a promising methylxanthine derivative for the treatment of asthma and chronic obstructive pulmonary disease." Expert Opin Pharmacother. 2009 Oct;10(14):2343-56; "Doxofylline ... has recently drawn attention because of its better safety profile and similar efficacy over the most widely prescribed analogue, theophylline, indicated for asthma and chronic obstructive pulmonary disease. ... In a relatively large number of comparative studies, doxofylline is indicated to have less affinity for alpha(1) and alpha(2) receptors than theophylline. Unlike theophylline, **doxofylline does not antagonize calcium channels, nor does it interfere with the influx of calcium into the cells**, which probably reduces the cardiac side effects. Moreover, **it does not affect sleep rhythm, gastric secretions, heart rate and rhythm and CNS functioning.** ... However, **despite its superior safety and clinical efficacy, the potential of doxofylline has not been fully exploited.**"

Pardakhti A, Alavi SA, Kheshti NM, Eshaghi P, Safaeian L. "Effect of slow release pentoxifylline and captopril on delayed pulmonary complications of mustard gas in **animal models.**" Tanaffos. 2009; 8(1), 41-49; **"Pentoxifylline only resulted in decreased pulmonary inflammation without any effects on other indices.** On the other hand, increase in hydroxyproline content of the lung in the captopril group compared to controls showed that captopril had accelerated the process of fibrosis."

Lauterbach R, Szymura-Oleksiak J, Pawlik D, Warchoł J, Lisowska-Miszczyk I, Rytlewski K. "**Nebulized pentoxifylline for prevention of bronchopulmonary dysplasia in very low birth weight infants**: a pilot clinical study." J Matern Fetal Neonatal Med. 2006 Jul;19(7):433-8.

Lauterbach R, Pawlik D, Zembala M, Szymura-Oleksiak J, Lisowska-Miszczyk I, Kowalczyk D, Bury J. "Pentoxyfylline [sic] in the prevention and treatment of chronic lung disease." Acta Paediatr Suppl. 2004 Feb;93(444):20-2.

Featherston RL, Chambers DJ, Kelly FJ. "Comparison of phosphodiesterase inhibitors of differing isoenzyme selectivity added to St. Thomas' Hospital Cardioplegic Solution used for hypothermic preservation of **rat** lungs." Am. J. Respir. Crit. Care Med. 2000 Sep;162(3):850-6; **Of the selective agents examined, those inhibiting the PDE IV isoenzyme subtype are the most effective. However, the apparent superiority of the nonselective agent [pentoxifylline] ... merits further investigation.**"

Entzian P, Schlaak M, Seitzer U, Acil Y, Ernst M, Zabel P. "Pentoxifylline inhibits the fibrogenic activity of pleural effusions and transforming growth factor-b." Mediators of Inflammation. 1997;6:119-126; "...49 consecutive patients suffering from non-carcinomatous pleurisy. ... we searched for **alternatives to steroid administration** and found evidence that elevating intracellular cAMP, eg with pentoxifylline, might be a promising approach. ... **pentoxifylline inhibits the effect of transforming growth factor-b [TFG-b] on fibrogenesis.** ... **pentoxifylline ... inhibits not only inflammatory mediators (as do corticosteroids) but fibrogenesis as well.** ... In conclusion, ... pentoxifylline – might be effective in prevention and therapy, not only of pleural fibrosis but of other fibrosing disorders as well. ... We feel that sufficient evidence now exists to propose pentoxifylline for a prospective therapeutic intervention study in human disease."

Aronoff SC, Quinn FJ Jr, Carpenter LS, Novick WJ Jr. "Effects of pentoxifylline on sputum neutrophil elastase and pulmonary function in **patients with cystic fibrosis**: preliminary observations." J Pediatr. 1994 Dec;125(6 Pt 1):992-7 [used pentoxifylline 1,600 mg/day]. [note that the dose used was four-thirds of the more commonly used dose]

MUSCLE & BLOOD FLOW DISORDERS (INCLUDING CLAUDICATION)

The abstracts listed below note the ability of pentoxifylline to improve muscle and other organ functions – apparently by enhancing oxygenation and reducing inflammation. Athletes seem to have paid more attention to this than have physicians.

Słoczyńska K, Kózka M, Pękala E, Marchewka A, Marona H. "In vitro effect of pentoxifylline and lisofylline on deformability and aggregation of red blood cells from healthy subjects and patients with chronic venous disease." Acta Biochim Pol. 2013;60(1):129-35.; "... **LSF [lisofylline] may contribute to the in vivo hemorheological effects of pentoxifylline.** On the other hand, **there was no significant effect of LSF on aggregation of RBC in vitro. Hence, LSF has no contribution to this particular**

61

effect of PTX [pentoxifylline]. ..."

Baykara M, Atabek ME, Eklioglu BS, Kurtoglu S. "Pentoxifylline treatment for protecting diabetic retinopathy in children with type 1 diabetes." J Pediatr Endocrinol Metab. 2013;26(1-2):19-24; "...56 type 1 [child] diabetic patients. ... were matched first in terms of age, diabetes duration, then one individual within each pair was randomized into a pentoxifylline group and a control group. Pentoxifylline was administered for 6 months. ... **In the pentoxifylline group there was a significant reduction in systolic blood pressure, diastolic blood pressure, microalbuminuria and an increase in HDL level.** Conclusion: Our results suggest that **pentoxifylline may have a protective action for diabetic retinopathy and might modulate risk factors for atherosclerosis in type 1 diabetes.**"

Gan EY, Tang MB, Tan SH, Chua SH, Tan AW. "A ten-year retrospective study on livedo vasculopathy in Asian patients." Ann Acad Med Singapore. 2012 Sep;41(9):400-6; "... a retrospective analysis of all patients [70] diagnosed with **LV [livedo vasculopathy] [painful leg ulcers]** from 1997 to 2007 at our centre. ... In 49 patients who achieved remission, 55% required combination therapy, most commonly with colchicine, pentoxifylline and prednisolone. In those treated successfully with monotherapy, colchicine was effective in 59% followed by prednisolone (17.5%), pentoxifylline (17.5%) and aspirin (6%). Mean follow-up period was 50 months. ... [while not the main point of this article, it is notable that **pentoxifylline worked as well as the less safe prednisolone** – and certainly remains a far safer option than colchicine]

Lauterbach R, Rytlewski K, Pawlik D, Hurkała J, Wójtowicz A, Bręborowicz G, Szymankiewicz M. "Effect of Pentoxifylline, administered in Preterm Labour, on the Foetal-Placental Circulation and Neonatal Outcome. A Randomized, Prospective Pilot Study." Basic Clin Pharmacol Toxicol. 2012 Apr;110(4):342-6; "... Pentoxifylline was given as a supplement to standard tocolytic therapy in a group of 43 patients ... as an intravenous infusion and oral supplementation in a total dosage of 800 mg/day. The drug was administered within three weeks after admission. No pentoxifylline was given in the control group (53 patients). … **The risk of severe neonatal complications was significantly lower in the pentoxifylline group** (p=0.026). **Pentoxifylline changed foetal-placental blood circulation in patients with threatened preterm labour and improved neonatal outcome**. [note that the dose used was two-thirds of the more commonly used dose]

O'Donnell TF Jr, Balk EM. "The need for an Intersociety Consensus Guideline for **venous ulcer**." J Vasc Surg. 2011 Sep 9; "Fourteen **guidelines** were identified, of which 13 were evidence-based … . **80% advocated pentoxifylline** …."

Atabek ME, Kurtoglu S, Selver B, Baykara M. "Effectiveness of pentoxifylline on the cross-sectional area of intima media thickness and functions of the common carotid artery in adolescents with type 1 diabetes." J Pediatr Endocrinol Metab. 2011;24(11-12):945-51; "… 56 type 1 diabetic patients. … matched first in terms of age, diabetes duration, major cardiovascular risk factors, including anthropometric and metabolic parameters as well as ultrasonographic measurements, then one individual within each pair randomized into a pentoxifylline group and a placebo (control) group (ie, 32 on pentoxifylline group and 24 on placebo). Pentoxifylline was administered for 6 months. … the pentoxifylline treatment group had significantly higher values than the controls for CSA-IMT [cross-sectional area of intima media thickness]… and for DWS [diastolic wall stress]…. Our preliminary results **suggest that pentoxifylline has an antiatherogenic action and might modulate risk factors for atherosclerosis in type 1 diabetes**."

Gohel MS, Davies AH. "Pharmacological treatment in patients with C4, C5, and C6 venous disease." Phebology. 2010 Oct:25 Suppl 1:35-41; "In prospective randomized studies, MPFF (Daflon), other flavonoid derivatives, and **pentoxifylline** have **demonstrated clinical benefits in patients with C4-C6 venous disease**" [C4 = has cutaneous & subcutaneous changes, C5 = has healed ulcers , C6 = has active ulcers].

"Professional Monograph (FDA): Cilostazol (Mylan Pharmaceuticals).

2010 Jul; "is extensively metabolized by hepatic cytochrome P-450 enzymes, mainly 3A4, and, to a lesser extent, 2C19.... Cilostazol and its active metabolites accumulate about 2-fold with chronic administration and reach steady-state blood levels within a few days. http://www.drugs.com/pro/cilostazol.html#ixzz13OBTbtfx .

[cilostazol frequently is marketed as an alternative to pentoxifylline – but **pentoxifylline does not have cytochrome P-450 interaction & does not accumulate** – both of these issues having to do with increased toxicity]

Committee on Social Security Cardiovascular Disability Criteria, Board on the Health of Select Populations & Institute of Medicine. Cardiovascular Disability: Updating the Social Security Listings. Washington, DC: The National Academies Press, 2010; pp.172, 185. [re **pentoxifylline has been recognized as for "leg pain" beyond "intermittent claudication"**]

Superhuman Gear; http://superhumangear.blogspot.com/2010/10/pentoxifylline-trental-for-flexible.html; see also Anemia Patient Group http://anemiapatientgroup.blogspot.com/2010_01_01_archive.html, which further specifies that "Pentoxifylline is supplied for laboratory research use only and not for human consumption"; both sites were accessed on 15-NOV-10. Pentoxifylline is easily available on the web, and a much-cited article is the following: Wood SC, Appenzeller O, Greene ER, Eldridge M. "Arterial oxygen saturation: effects of altitude and pentoxifylline." J Wilderness Med. 1992 Aug;3(3):250-255; "... **Pentoxifylline, a rheologically active drug, increases maximum heart rate at high altitude.** ... Twelve subjects were tested at 2,100 m, 2,730 m, and 4,600 m altitude. In a double blind protocol, 6 subjects took pentoxifylline (1,200 mg per day) each day for five weeks before and during the study. Control subjects ($n = 6$) took a placebo. The most important finding was **a significantly higher resting arterial saturation at 4,600 m in the [mountain climbing] subjects taking pentoxifylline** (80.7% versus 75.4% in the control group). Possible mechanisms of this action of pentoxifylline include improved pulmonary gas exchange." Professor Stephen C. Wood, director of the Mountain Research

Foundation [and an editor with Robert C. Roach of Sports and Exercise Medicine (Lung Biology in Health and Disease, Volume 76). New York: Marcel Dekker, 1994] is world-renowned for his physiologic investigations in Ladakh and Sikkim. Intriguingly, the US government-sponsored website, PubMed Health ["Last reviewed: September 1, 2008"], notes that **pentoxifylline also is used for "high-altitude sickness"** – even though there are no double-blind, randomized, placebo-controlled, multicenter studies of this – beyond Professor Wood's article that is much-cited by bloggers. **The ability of pentoxifylline to reduce muscle wasting**, especially in rats, also is much referenced on the web by "body builders," as **a means to reduce steroid use** – with the following being the two most relevant (and encouraging) articles: von Haehling S, Lainscak M, Springer J, Anker SD. "Cardiac cachexia: a systematic overview." Pharmacol Ther. 2009 Mar;121(3):227-52; "... The mechanisms of wasting in different body compartments are described. ... Other drug classes of interest comprise angiotensin-converting enzyme inhibitors, beta-blockers, anabolic steroids, beta-adrenergic agonists, anti-inflammatory substances, statins, thalidomide, proteasome inhibitors, and **pentoxifylline**." Combaret L, Rallière C, Taillandier D, Tanaka K, Attaix D. "Manipulation of the ubiquitin-proteasome pathway in cachexia: pentoxifylline suppresses the activation of 20S and 26S proteasomes in muscles from tumor-bearing rats." Mol Biol Rep. 1999 Apr;26(1-2):95-101; "... We have shown here that **a daily administration of PTX [pentoxifylline] prevents muscle atrophy and suppresses increased protein breakdown** in Yoshida sarcoma-bearing **rats** by inhibiting the activation of a nonlysosomal, $Ca(2+)$-independent proteolytic pathway. ... This is the first demonstration of a pharmacological manipulation of the ubiquitin-proteasome pathway in cachexia with **a drug which is well tolerated in humans. Overall, the data suggest that PTX [pentoxifylline] can prevent muscle wasting ... ."**

Laczy B, Cseh J, Mohás M, Markó L, Tamaskó M, Koszegi T, Molnár GA, Wagner Z, Wagner L, Wittmann I. "Effects of pentoxifylline and pentosan polysulphate combination therapy on **diabetic neuropathy** in type 2 diabetes mellitus." Acta Diabetol. 2009 Jun;46(2):105-11; "... Patients in Verum [active treatment] group (n = 77) received PF-PPS infusions **[pentoxifylline + pentosan]** (100-100 mg/day) for 5 days. [Pentosan is a semisynthetic pentasaccharide heparinoid.] Control diabetics (placebo group; n = 12) were given only saline infusions. Specialized cardiovascular autonomic reflex tests, [and] vibration threshold values ... were assessed before and after therapy. In Verum group, **autonomic score, indicating the severity of cardiac autonomic dysfunction, decreased after therapy** ... . Of the reflexes, **deep breath and handgrip tests also improved after therapy** ... . **Vibration threshold values, an indicator of the loss of sensory nerve function, were increased after therapy** ... . In conclusion, **short-term PF-PPS [pentoxifylline + pentosan] therapy was effective on cardiovascular autonomic function and vibration perception** ... .

Noaimi AA, Fadheel BM. "Treatment of perniosis [pernio; chilblains; inflammation secondary to damp cold] with oral pentoxyfylline in comparison with oral prednisolone plus topical clobetasol ointment in Iraqi patients." Saudi Med J. 2008 Dec;29(12):1762-4; "...In group A [glucocorticoids], 11 patients completed the treatment course, and only 3 27.2% patients showed good improvement and complete cure after 2 weeks. In group B [pentoxifylline], 9 patients completed the regime, and 5 55.5% patients showed good improvement, in which symptoms disappeared and lesions resolved after 2 weeks. ... **Pentoxyfylline was shown to be an effective and safe drug for treatment of perniosis [chilblains], and superior to oral plus topical glucocorticoids** $p<0.05$."

Hödl S. ["Treatment of freezing injury"][article in German; abstract in English is per www.pubmed.gov]. Wien Med Wochenschr. 2005 Apr;155(7-8):199-203; "**Pentoxifyllin [sic] is considered to lower pathologically increased levels of fibrinogen**"; "**may improve tissue perfusion and therefore tissue damage caused by frostbite can be limited.**"

Pipinos II, Boska MD, Shepard AD, Anagnostopoulos PV, Katsamouris A. "Pentoxifylline reverses oxidative mitochondrial defect in claudicating skeletal muscle." J Surg Res. 2002 Feb;102(2):126-32; "significant improvement in mitochondrial function with pentoxifylline";

"Pentoxifylline improves the mitochondriopathy of claudicating muscle, producing the most improvement in limbs with the worse baseline mitochondrial function."

Sanganalmath SK, Barta J, Takeda N, Kumamoto H, Dhalla NS. "Antiplatelet therapy mitigates cardiac remodeling and dysfunction in congestive heart failure due to myocardial infarction." Can J Physiol Pharmacol. 2008 Apr;86(4):180-9; " ... CIL [cilostazol] increased the incidence of ventricular arrhythmias and the mean number of episodes in infarcted animals [rats]. Mortality during the treatment period was ... increased by 10% with CIL, but these changes were not significant statistically. ..." [compared to the beneficial effects of pentoxifylline in congestive heart failure; cilostazol frequently is marketed as an alternative to pentoxifylline]

Food and Drug Administration (US). "Professional Monograph (FDA): Pentoxifylline (Mylan Pharmaceuticals). 2006 Dec; "There is no evidence of accumulation or enzyme induction (Cytochrome P450) following multiple oral doses [of pentoxifylline]."
http://www.drugs.com/pro/pentoxifylline.html#ixzz13OBkKgcM ;

Tjon JA, Riemann LE. "Treatment of Intermittent Claudication: Pentoxifylline and Cilostazol." American Journal of Health-System Pharmacy. 2001;58(6):485-93 [an excellent comparing and contrasting of the two medications; as noted above, pentoxifylline is far safer; the two medications, however, can be used together].

Lee TM, Su SF, Tsai CH, Lee YT, Wang SS. "Differential effects of cilostazol and pentoxifylline on vascular endothelial growth factor in patients with intermittent claudication." Clin Sci. 2001; 101, 305–311; "... Circulating VEGF levels were increased (from 116^329 to 169^345 pg/ml; $P^-0.002$) ... in those patients treated with cilostazol that did not have diabetes mellitus. ... However, **pentoxifylline did not affect VEGF [vascular endothelial growth factor] levels, although a similar improvement in maximal walking distance was achieved.**" [an obvious question – whether the increased VEGF seen with cilostazol increases angiogenesis – is argued from both sides in the following two articles:] Mendes JB, Campos PP, Rocha MA, Andrade SP. "Cilostazol and pentoxifylline decrease angiogenesis, inflammation, and fibrosis in sponge-induced intraperitoneal adhesion in mice." Life Sci. 2009 Apr 10;84(15-16):537-43; "...VEGF levels were also decreased by approximately 40% ... ." Otagiri A, Matsushita S, Sakakibara Y. http://www.sciencedirect.com/science?_ob=ArticleURL&_udi=B6T99-4VM446B-1&_user=10&_coverDate=04%2F10%2F2009&_rdoc=1&_fmt=full&_orig=search&_origin=search&_cdi=5109&_sort=d&_docanchor=&view=c&_searchStrId=1582642689&_rerunOrigin=google&_acct=C000050221&_version=1&_urlVersion=0&_userid=10&md5=d24b152547613d1f8776ea8e8b123c65&searchtype=a "Effect of PDIII inhibitor (Cilostazol) on ischemic angiogenesis in diabetic mice." FASEB J. 2009 Apr 23 (Meeting Abstract Supplement) 625.4; "... Cilostazol enhanced angiogenesis in diabetic ischemic limb. It is not due to the involvement of bone-marrow derived EPCs, but may due to enhanced eNOS expression ... ."

De Backer TL, Vander Stichele RH, Van Bortel LM. "Letter regarding article, 'Oral buflomedil in the prevention of cardiovascular events in patients with peripheral arterial obstructive disease: a randomized, placebo-controlled, 4-year study'.". Circulation. 2008 Sep 2;118(10):e151; "...the LIMB trial provides limited evidence for a clinically meaningful benefit of buflomedil, both with regard to hard and soft cardiovascular end points and with regard to symptomatic improvement in walking distance. However, we would like to add information on the safety issue. The potential toxicity of the product, stemming from a series of case reports, is worrisome. In 2005, the French National Commission for Pharmacovigilance conducted a historical review of case series of voluntary and involuntary (such as in patients with renal insufficiency) overdose with neurological (primarily myoclonic twitches and convulsions) and cardiovascular adverse reactions (mainly arrhythmias and cardiac arrest), with lethal dosages starting at 5 to 6 g. The French authorities decided in 2006 to withdraw the 600-mg and 300-mg formulations of buflomedil because of its narrow therapeutic margin and to impose major restrictions in the labeling. Similar actions were taken in other countries where buflomedil is marketed. In our opinion, **the balance between benefit and risk for buflomedil is unsatisfactory** and insufficient evidence exists to integrate buflomedil routinely into the guidelines for treatment of intermittent claudication." [while buflomedil (4-pyrrolidin-1-yl-1-(2,4,6-trimethoxyphenyl)butan-1-one) has never been approved for marketing in the United States, it has enjoyed waves of popularity elsewhere – as an alternative to pentoxifylline – and thus is mentioned here; it is notably less safe than pentoxifylline]

Sacerdote A. "Treatment of homozygous sickle cell disease with pentoxifylline." J Natl Med Assoc. 1999 Aug;91(8):466-70: "... sustained symptomatic and hematologic improvement in a 21-year-old woman with **homozygous sickle cell (ss) disease** during treatment with pentoxifylline, 400 mg three times daily after meals. **Pain crises decreased from six to zero per year, hemoglobin level rose from 8.4 g/dL to 11.4 g/dL, hematocrit rose from 24.8% to 34.8%**, lactate dehydrogenase level decreased from 375 IU/L to 322 IU/L, and total bilirubin level decreased from 1.8 mg/dL to 1.6 mg/dL. **Mean corpuscular hemoglobin increased from 21.6 pg to 30 pg** and **mean corpuscular hemoglobin concentration increased from 24.1 g/dL to 34.5 g/dL**. These changes were sustained for seven years except for a brief self-imposed hiatus in therapy during which period a pain crisis occurred. ..."

Poflee VW, Gupta OP, Jain AP, Jajoo UN. "Haemorheological treatment of painful sickle cell crises. Use of pentoxifylline." J Assoc Physicians India. 1991 Aug;39(8):608-9; "... pentoxifylline ... was tried in nine patients with **painful vaso-occlusive crises**. Another nine matched patients served as control. While no patient in the control group improved, **five patients in the pentoxifylline group responded favourably within 48 hours. ...**"

BONE & JOINT (ORTHOPEDIC & RHEUMATOLOGIC) DISORDERS

The abstracts listed below focus on skeletal and joint issues that tend to be hard to heal.

Erken HY, Burc H, Aydogan M. "The Effect of Pentoxifylline on Spinal Fusion: An Experimental Study in Rabbits." Spine (Phila Pa 1976). 2014. 39(11):E676-E683; "… Randomized, double-blinded, **animal model**. … Conclusions. The differences between groups was statistically significant in terms of radiological fusion grading, biomechanical testing, volume of the fusion mass, and percentage of trabecular bone area. These **results suggest that PTX [pentoxifylline] may have a beneficial effect on spinal fusion**.

Mohammed SI, Gorial FI, Majeed IA. "Pentoxifylline as Adjuvant Therapy to Etanercept in Patients with Moderately to Highly Active Rheumatoid Arthritis." Am J Pharmacol Sci. 2013;1(4):61-66; [40 of 49 randomized patients nonresponsive to 4 months of etanercept completed 8 weeks of pentoxifylline 400 mg bid] "... **PTX [pentoxifylline] significantly decreased pro-inflammatory markers (TNF, hsCRP), duration of morning stiffness, and cardiovascular risk**. This may suggest that **PTX pentoxifylline could be a promising and useful strategy to reduce the systemic inflammation and cardiovascular morbidity and mortality observed in RA [rheumatoid arthritis] patients**."

Delanian S, Chatel C, Porcher R, Depondt J, Lefaix JL. "Complete restoration of refractory mandibular osteoradionecrosis by prolonged treatment with **a pentoxifylline-tocopherol-clodronate combination** (PENTOCLO): A phase II trial." Int J Radiat Oncol Biol Phys. 2010 Jul 15; "Long-term PENTOCLO treatment **is effective, safe, and curative for refractory ORN [osteoradionecrosis] and induces mucosal and bone healing with significant symptom improvement**."

Sugama R, Koike T, Imai Y, Nomura-Furuwatari C, Takaoka K. "Bone morphogenetic protein activities are enhanced by 3',5'-cyclic adenosine monophosphate through suppression of [smooth muscle actin] Smad6 expression in osteoprogenitor cells." Bone. 2006 Feb;38(2):206-14; " …**pentoxifyline (PeTx), a nonspecific inhibitor of phosphodiesterase**

(PDE), and rolipram, a PDE-4-specific inhibitor, enhance BMP-4-induced osteogenic [bone-forming] differentiation of mesenchymal cells ... ."

Usha PR, Naidu MUR, Datla R. "Clinical efficacy and tolerability evaluation of pentoxifylline in **rheumatoid arthritis**: A double-blind, randomised, placebo-controlled study." Clin Drug Investig. 2002;22(5):329-39; " ... 53 patients (28 receiving pentoxifylline and 25 placebo) were enrolled in the study. ... **Both tender and swollen joint count reduced significantly** from 16.8 ± 2.6 to 12.7 ± 3.4 and 9.5 ± 4.4, and from 6.5 ± 1.1 to 4.3 ± 1.3 and 3.7 ± 1.6 after 12 and 24 weeks, respectively, with pentoxifylline. Placebo did not decrease the above parameters. ... **A statistically significant decrease in erythrocyte sedimentation rate, rheumatoid factor immunoglobulin M, C-reactive protein and malondialdehyde was observed with pentoxifylline** compared with placebo. **The response rate was 57% with pentoxifylline compared with 19% with placebo. ...**"

Rawadi G, Ferrer C, Spinella-Jaegle S, Roman-Roman S, Bouali Y, Baron R. "1-(5-oxohexyl)-3,7-Dimethylxanthine, a phosphodiesterase inhibitor, activates MAPK cascades and promotes osteoblast differentiation by a mechanism independent of PKA activation (pentoxifylline promotes osteoblast differentiation)." Endocrinology. 2001 Nov;142(11):4673-82; "... **PeTx [pentoxifylline] is able to enhance [bone morphogenic protein] BMP-2-induced [smooth muscle actin D] Smad1 transcriptional activity.** ... PeTx induced the activation of [extracellular-regulated kinases] ERK1/2 and p38 kinase pathways independently of the activation of PKA [protein kinase A]. Selective inhibitors of these MAPK [mitogen-activated protein kinases] cascades prevented the induction of osteoblastic markers in cells treated with PeTx, suggesting that the activation of these two pathways plays a role in **the effect of PeTx [pentoxifylline] on osteoblastic [bone-cell] differentiation.**"

Ishii O, Yamada H, Ohya S, Moriuchi E, Kase C, Ichikawa Y, Yamasaki K. ["Remission induction after pentoxifylline treatment in a patient with rheumatoid arthritis"] [article in Japanese; abstract in English is per www.pubmed.gov]. Ryumachi. 1997 Dec;37(6):810-5; "Discontinuation of POF [pentoxifylline] resulted in rapid exacerbation of RA. **POF [pentoxifylline] was restarted and the patient showed complete recovery from arthritis with normalization of ESR [erythrocyte sedimentation rate] within 3 months and was maintained a complete remission for another 1 year**. This case further supports **a potential antirheumatic effect of POF [pentoxifylline] on some patients with RA [rheumatoid arthritis]**."

BRAIN (PSYCHIATRIC/ NEUROLOGIC) DISORDERS (INCLUDING PAIN)

> *The abstracts listed below hint at the multitude of neuropsychiatric conditions that might respond positively to pentoxifylline. [Parkinson's disorder might be made worse by pentoxifylline.] Thus far, most of the research has been conducted in non-humans or has been incidental. Clearly, helping patients who have various forms of brain damage or deterioration is a challenge that must be surmounted. The present author is a psychiatrist, but many who are not could argue that this is the most exciting part of this monograph*

Heckman PR, Blokland A, Ramaekers J, Prickaerts J. "PDE and cognitive processing: beyond the memory domain." Neurobiol Learn Mem. Mar 2015;119:108-122; "... **attention, information filtering** (sensory- and sensorimotor gating) **and response inhibition** (drug-induced hyperlocomotion). ... Here we discuss experimental studies and the potential beneficial effects of PDE-I [phosphodiesterase inhibitor] drugs on these cognitive domains ... . Overall, **PDE4 [phosphodiesterase 4] [eg, what pentoxifylline inhibits] seems to be the most promising target for all domains discussed in this review**."

Ahmad M, Abu-Taweel GM, Aboshaiqah AE, Ajarem JS. "The effects of quinacrine, proglumide, and pentoxifylline on seizure activity, cognitive deficit, and oxidative stress in [adult] **rat** lithium-pilocarpine model of status epilepticus." Oxid Med Cell Longev. 2014;2014: Article ID 630509,

11 pages; "... Quinacrine (Qcn), proglumide (Pgm), and **pentoxifylline (Ptx) administered to animals before inducing SE [status epilepticus], were significantly effective in ameliorating the seizure activities, cognitive dysfunctions, and cerebral OS [oxidative stress].** The findings suggest that all the drugs were effective in the order of Ptx < Pgm < Qcn indicating that these drugs are **potentially antiepileptic as well as antioxidant ....**"

Gough B, Pereira FC, Fontes Ribeiro CA, Ali SF, Binienda ZK. "Propentophylline increases striatal dopamine release but dampens methamphetamine-induced dopamine dynamics: A microdialysis study." Neurochem Int. 2014 Jul 15;76C:109-113; "... **propentofylline (PPF), an atypical methylxanthine, can suppress the rewarding effects of methamphetamine (METH) in mice.** ... PPF ... attenuates METH-induced striatal DA release and metabolism."

Blednov YA, Benavidez JM, Black M, Harris RA. "Inhibition of phosphodiesterase 4 reduces ethanol intake and preference in C57BL/6J **mice.**" Front Neurosci. 2014 May 27;8:129; "... Our results provide novel evidence for a selective role of PDE4 in regulating ethanol drinking in mice. We suggest that **inhibition of PDE4 [phosphodiesterase 4] [eg, what pentoxifylline inhibits] may be an unexplored target for medication development to reduce excessive alcohol consumption.**"

Reissner KJ, Brown RM, Spencer S, Tran PK, Thomas CA, Kalivas PW. "Chronic Administration of the Methylxanthine Propentofylline Impairs Reinstatement to Cocaine by a GLT-1-Dependent Mechanism." Neuropsychopharmacology. 2014 Jan;39(2):499-506; "...We found that 7 days of **chronic (but not acute) administration of PPF [propentofylline] significantly decreased both cue- and cocaine-induced reinstatement of cocaine seeking [in rats].** ... PPF restored the cocaine-induced decrease in GLT-1 [an astroglial glutamate transporter] in the accumbens core; ... we found that restored transporter expression was necessary for PPF to inhibit cue-primed cocaine seeking. These findings indicate that **modulating glial physiology with atypical xanthine derivatives like PPF [propentofylline] is a potential avenue**

for developing new medications for cocaine abuse ... ."

Chiu S, Gericke N, Farina-Woodbury M, Badmaev V, Raheb H, Terpstra K, Antongiorgi J, Bureau Y, Cernovsky Z, Hou J, Sanchez V, Williams M, Copen J, Husni M, Goble L. "Proof-of-Concept Randomized Controlled Study of Cognition Effects of the Proprietary Extract Sceletium tortuosum (Zembrin) Targeting Phosphodiesterase-4 in Cognitively Healthy Subjects: Implications for Alzheimer's Dementia." Evid Based Complement Alternat Med. 2014;2014:682014; "... **In the recombinant PDE4 [phosphodiesterase 4] in vitro assay, [the herb]** *Sceletium tortuosum* **(Zembrin) selectively inhibited PDE-4 [as does pentoxifylline].** [In a randomized placebo-controlled 3-week cross-over design,] "... **Zembrin enhanced cognition in the domains of executive functioning and cognitive flexibility in healthy subjects. ...**"

Richter W, Menniti FS, Zhang HT, Conti M. "PDE4 [phosphodiesterase 4] as a target for cognition enhancement." Expert Opin Ther Targets. 2013 Sep;17(9):1011-27; "... **PAN-selective PDE4 [phosphodiesterase 4] inhibitors [eg, pentoxifylline] exert a number of memory- and cognition-enhancing effects and have neuroprotective and neuroregenerative properties in preclinical models.** ... The PDE4 family comprises four genes, PDE4A-D, each expressed as multiple variants. ... Thus, targeting specific PDE4 subtypes, as well as splicing variants or conformational states, represents a promising strategy to separate the therapeutic benefits from the side effects of PAN-PDE4 inhibitors."

Mohamed T, Osman W, Tin G, Rao PP. "Selective inhibition of human acetylcholinesterase by xanthine derivatives: in vitro inhibition and molecular modeling investigations." Bioorg Med Chem Lett. 2013 Aug 1;23(15):4336-41; "... we investigated the cholinesterase inhibition by the xanthine derivatives caffeine, pentoxifylline, and propentofylline. Among them, **propentofylline was the most potent AChE [acetyl cholinesterase] inhibitor** (hAChE IC_{50}=6.40 μM). ... In summary, our study has important implications in the development of novel caffeine derivatives as selective AChE inhibitors with **potential application as**

cognitive enhancers and to treat various forms of dementia."

Zhang, Jin; Wu, Dan; Xie, Cheng; Wang, Huan; Wang, Wei; Zhang, Hui; Liu, Rui; Xu, Li-Xian; Mei, Xiao-Peng. "Tramadol and Propentofylline Coadministration Exerted Synergistic Effects on **Rat** Spinal Nerve Ligation-Induced Neuropathic Pain." PLoS ONE. Aug 2013;8(8):1; "...**Tramadol and propentofylline coadministration exerted a more potent effect in a synergistic and dose dependent manner than the intrathecal administration of either drug alone. ...**"

Almond M. "Depression and inflammation: Examining the link." Current Psychi. June 2013;12(6):25-32 [excellent summary review].

O'Donovan A, Rush G, Hoatam G, Hughes BM, McCrohan A, Kelleher C, O'Farrelly C, Malone KM. "Suicidal ideation is associated with elevated inflammation in patients with major depressive disorder." Depress Anxiety. 2013 Apr;30(4):307-14; "...we measured inflammatory markers in patients with MDD [major depressive disorder] with and without high levels of suicidal ideation and in nondepressed controls (N = 124). ... A composite score including the inflammatory markers tumor necrosis factor-α (TNF-α), interleukin-6 (IL-6), interleukin-10 (IL-10), and C-reactive protein (CRP) was used as an inflammatory index. ... Patients with MDD and **high suicidal ideation had significantly higher inflammatory index scores** than both controls ... and patients with MDD and lower suicidal ideation .... In contrast, patients with lower suicidal ideation were not significantly different from controls ...." [pentoxifylline lowers tumor necrosis factor-α (TNF-α), interleukin-6 (IL-6), and C-reactive protein (CRP) – 3 of the 4 inflammation markers noted above]

Raison CL, Rutherford RE, Woolwine BJ, Shuo C, Schettler P, Drake DF, Haroon E, Miller AH. "A randomized controlled trial of the tumor necrosis factor antagonist infliximab for treatment-resistant depression: the role of baseline inflammatory biomarkers." JAMA Psychiatry. 2013 Jan;70(1):31-41; "...**TNF antagonism** does not have generalized efficacy in treatment-resistant depression but **may improve depressive symptoms in patients with high baseline inflammatory biomarkers.**"

Godlevsky LS, Drozdova GA, Kobolev EV, Mustyatsa VF, Polyasnyi VA. "Pentoxifylline potentiates antiepileptic activity of diazepam on the model of treatment-resistant focal epilepsy." [article in English, Russian; abstract in English is per www.pubmed.gov] Bull Exp Biol Med. 2012 Dec;154(3):326-328; "...Kindling-syndrome was modeled in male Wistar **rats** using repeated corazole administration ... . The effects of pentoxifylline (25 and 100 mg/kg intraperitoneally) and diazepam (0.05 and 1 mg/kg intraperitoneally) were studied in 3 weeks after kindling development ... . **An anticonvulsant effect of combined treatment with diazepam and pentoxifylline, in the doses ineffective if administered separately ..., was demonstrated.**"

Stewart JC. "Anti-INFLammatory to Address Mood and Endothelial Dysfunction (INFLAMED)." ClinicalTrials.gov identifier: NCT01625845; study start date: June 2012; "...to examine whether adding an anti-inflammatory medication (pentoxifylline [400 mg po tid for 12 weeks]) to standard depression treatment (cognitive-behavioral therapy) improves both depressive symptoms and endothelial dysfunction, a sign of early cardiovascular disease. ..."

Bah TM, Kaloustian S, Rousseau G, Godbout R. "Pretreatment with pentoxifylline has antidepressant-like effects in a rat model of acute myocardial infarction." Behav Pharmacol. 2011 Oct 1; "...We conclude that **PTX [pentoxifylline] administration significantly reverses the depressive-like behaviour seen after MI [myocardial infarction] in rats.**"

Janelidze S, Mattei D, Westrin A, Träskman-Bendz L, Brundin L. "Cytokine levels in the blood may distinguish suicide attempters from depressed patients." Brain Behav Immun. 2011 Feb;25(2):335-9. "...Plasma interleukin (IL)-2, IL-6 and tumor necrosis factor (TNF)-α were measured in 47 suicide attempters, 17 non-suicidal depressed patients and 16 healthy controls. ... **We found increased levels of IL-6 and TNF-α as well as decreased IL-2 concentrations in suicide attempters compared to non-suicidal depressed patients and healthy**

controls. [pentoxifylline lowers both IL-6 and TNF-α] The results were adjusted for potential confounders of cytokine expression, such as age, sex, body mass index (BMI), degree of depression, anxiety, personality disturbance, abuse and type of medication. These results demonstrate for the first time that suicidal patients display a distinct peripheral blood cytokine profile compared to non-suicidal depressed patients. Thus, **our study provides further support for a role of inflammation in the pathophysiology of suicidality.**"

Wager-Smith K, Markou A. "Depression: A repair response to stress-induced neuronal microdamage that can grade into a chronic neuroinflammatory condition?" Neurosci Biobehav Rev. 2011 Jan;35(3):742-64; "**In this model, a stressful life event leads to microdamage in the brain. This damage triggers an injury repair response consisting of a neuroinflammatory phase to clear cellular debris, and a spontaneous tissue regeneration phase involving neurotrophins and neurogenesis. During healing, released inflammatory mediators trigger sickness behavior and psychological pain via mechanisms similar to those that produce physical pain during wound healing. The depression remits if the neuronal injury repair process resolves successfully.** Importantly, however, **the acute psychological pain and neuroinflammation often transition to chronicity and develop into pathological depressive states.**"

Xu Y, Zhang HT, O'Donnell JM "Phosphodiesterases in the central nervous system: implications in mood and cognitive disorders." Handb Exp Pharmacol. 2011;(204):447-85; "… Since PDEs have been shown to play distinct roles in processes of emotion and related learning and memory processes, **selective PDE [phosphodiesterase] inhibitors, by preventing the breakdown of cAMP and/or cGMP, modulate mood and related cognitive activity.** This review discusses the current state and future development in the burgeoning field of PDEs in the central nervous system. **It is becoming increasingly clear that PDE [phosphodiesterase] inhibitors have therapeutic potential for the treatment of neuropsychiatric disorders involving disturbances of mood, emotion, and cognition.**" [pentoxifylline primarily inhibits production of phosphodiesterase 4 – but somewhat inhibits production of phosphodiesterases 1, 2, 3, & 5]

Sweitzer S, De Leo J. "Propentofylline: glial modulation, neuroprotection, and alleviation of chronic pain." Handb Exp Pharmacol. 2011;(200):235-50 [entire issue also sold as Fredholm BB, editor. Methylxanthines. New York: Springer-Verlag, 2011]; "**Propentofylline has shown efficacy in preclinical models of stroke, opioid tolerance, and acute and chronic pain.** Clinically**, propentofylline has shown efficacy in degenerative and vascular dementia, and as a potential adjuvant treatment for schizophrenia and multiple sclerosis.** Possible mechanisms of action include a **direct glial modulation to decrease** a reactive phenotype, decrease glial production and release of **damaging proinflammatory factors**, and **enhancement of astrocyte-mediated glutamate clearance.**"

Jain KK. The handbook of neuroprotection. New York: Humana Press/ Springer, 2011; provides a concise summary: pp.32-33, "Propentofylline. This is **a neuroprotective glial cell modulator** .... by blocking adenosine transport and inhibition of cyclic adenosine monophosphate (cAMP) and cGMP-phosphodiesterase. ... **Propentoxifylline inhibits cytoxic functions of activated micoglia and also modulates astrocytic functions by stimulating nerve growth factor (NGF) synthesis and secretion.** ... Postischemic administration of Propentoxifylline increases adenosine levels in the brain, **reduces glutamate release, and improves glucose metabolism in all regions of the brain.**"

Clark IA, Alleva LM, Vissel B. "The roles of TNF in brain dysfunction and disease." Pharmacol Ther. 2010 Dec;128(3):519-48; "... Certain cytokines, the prototype being the highly pleiotropic TNF, have many homeostatic physiological roles, are involved in innate immunity, and cause inflammation when in excess. These cytokines have long been accepted to have central roles in the pathogenesis of systemic or local non-cerebral disease states, whether acute or chronic, and whether or not caused by infectious agents. ... As in other organs, excessive levels in brain are harmful .... Basic brain physiology is thus informing knowledge of the brain dysfunction that characterizes such apparently diverse states as Alzheimer's disease, trauma (mostly, but not only, to the brain), Parkinson's disease, and severe systemic infectious states, including malaria, sepsis, viral diseases and major depression. The implication is that **the anti-cytokine therapies now in use, typically directed at TNF, warrant testing in these diseases in circumstances in which the therapeutic agent enters the cerebrospinal fluid. ...**"

Swardfager W, Lanctôt K, Rothenburg L, Wong A, Cappell J, Herrmann N. "A meta-analysis of cytokines in Alzheimer's disease." Biol Psychiatry. 2010 Nov 15;68(10):930-41; "... Forty studies measuring peripheral blood cytokine concentrations and 14 measuring cerebrospinal fluid (CSF) cytokine concentrations were included. ... These results strengthen the clinical evidence that **AD [Alzheimer's disease] is accompanied by an inflammatory response, particularly higher peripheral concentrations of IL-6, TNF-α,** IL-1β, TGF-β, IL-12 and IL-18 and higher CSF concentrations of TGF-β. [pentoxifylline reduces IL-6 and TNF-α – 2 of the 7 inflammatory molecules mentioned here]

Pasco JA, Nicholson GC, Williams LJ, Jacka FN, Henry MJ, Kotowicz MA, Schneider HG, Leonard BE, Berk M. "Association of high-sensitivity C-reactive protein with de novo major depression." Br J Psychiatry. 2010 Nov;197(5):372-7; "... 1494 randomly selected women recruited at baseline during the period 1994-7, 822 were **followed for a decade** and provided measures of both exposure and outcome. Of these women, 644 (aged 20-84 years) had no prior history of depression at baseline and were eligible for analysis. ... During 5,827 person-years of follow-up, 48 cases of de novo major depressive disorder were identified. **The hazard ratio (HR) for depression increased by 44% for each standard deviation increase in log-transformed hsCRP [high sensitivity C-reactive protein]...** after adjusting for weight, smoking and use of non-steroidal anti-inflammatory drugs. Further adjustment for other lifestyle factors, medications and comorbidity failed to explain the observed increased risk for depression. ... **Serum hsCRP is an independent risk marker for de novo major depressive disorder in women. This supports an aetiological role for inflammatory activity in the pathophysiology of depression.**" [pentoxifylline reduces CRP (C-reactive protein)]

Kohgami S, Ogata T, Morino T, Yamamoto H, Schubert P. "Pharmacological shift of the ambiguous nitric oxide action from neurotoxicity to cyclic GMP-mediated protection." Neurol Res. 2010 Nov;32(9):938-44; "…using a newly developed nitric oxide-related injury model of cultured spinal cord neurons. … These results suggest that NO [nitric oxide] has an ambiguous action, ie, toxic by favoring the formation of, but protective by intracellular cyclic GMP [guanosine monophosphate] elevation which can be reinforced by PDE [phosphodiesterase] inhibition. Therefore, **PDE [phosphodiesterase] inhibitors, such as PPF [propentofylline], may be useful therapeutic drugs to limit oxidative neuronal damage in the central nervous system.**"

Chou RC. "Tumor Necrosis Factor Inhibition Reduces the Incidence of Alzheimer's Disease in Rheumatoid Arthritis Patients." American College of Rheumatology Annual Scientific Meeting 2010 Nov 8; "… 165 RA subjects with Alzheimer's dementia were compared to 1,383 RA controls without Alzheimer's dementia. … **those [rheumatoid arthritis patients] who received anti-TNF treatment had a 55 percent reduction in risk of developing Alzheimer's dementia**. This effect was not seen with other drugs used for treatment of RA, including sulfasalazine, prednisone and rituximab."
http://www.rheumatology.org/about/newsroom/2010/2010_anti_tnf_ther apies_for_rheumatoid_arthritis_could_reduce_alzheimers_risk.asp

Diniz BS, Teixeira AL, Ojopi EB, Talib LL, Mendonça VA, Gattaz WF, Forlenza OV. "Higher serum sTNFR1 level predicts conversion from mild cognitive impairment to Alzheimer's disease." J Alzheimers Dis. 2010 Oct 7; "… **Abnormal activation of TNF-α signaling system**, represented by increased expression of sTNFR1, **is associated with a higher risk of progression from MCI [mild cognitive impairment] to AD [Alzheimer's disease]**. [pentoxifylline reduces TNF-α]

Maes M. "Depression is an inflammatory disease, but cell-mediated immune activation is the key component of depression." Prog Neuropsychopharmacol Biol Psychiatry. 2010 Jun 20; "based on meta-analysis results - **depression is an inflammatory disorder because the plasma levels of two cytokines are increased, i.e. interleukin-(IL)-6 and tumor necrosis factor-alpha (TNF-alpha)**"; "inflammation and cell-mediated immune activation are key factors in depression." [pentoxifylline reduces interleukin-(IL)-6 and tumor necrosis factor-alpha (TNF-alpha)]

Hameed H, Hameed M, Christo PJ. "The effect of morphine on glial cells as a potential therapeutic target for pharmacological development of analgesic drugs." Curr Pain Headache Rep. 2010 Apr;14(2):96-104: that **pentoxifylline shows "promising profiles for providing significant relief from opioid side effects, while simultaneously potentiating opioid analgesia"; "pentoxifylline has been shown to attenuate neuropathic pain states and may also contribute to reduction of morphine-induced tolerance and reward."**

Alagiakrishnan K, Masaki K. "Vascular dementia: Treatment & medication." Medscape. 2010 Apr 02; referencing the "European Pentoxifylline Multi-Infarct Dementia (EPMID) Study Group." Eur Neurol. 1996;36(5):315-21.

Janssen DG, Caniato RN, Verster JC, Baune BT. "A psychoneuroimmunological review on cytokines involved in antidepressant treatment response." Hum Psychopharmacol. 2010 Apr;25(3):201 15; "systematically reviewed the scientific literature on the subject over the last 20 years"; "**Antidepressants appear to normalize serum levels of major inflammatory cytokines, including interleukin (IL)-1beta, IL-6, tumor necrosis factor alpha (TNF-alpha), and interferon gamma (IFN-gamma).** Antidepressants are postulated to modulate cytokine functioning through their effects on intracellular cyclic adenosyl monophosphate (cAMP), serotonin metabolism, the hypothalamo-pituitary-adrenocortical (HPA) axis or through a direct action on neurogenesis." [pentoxifylline reduces IL-6, tumor necrosis factor alpha (TNF-alpha) – 2 of the 4 inflammatory molecules mentioned]

Dubovsky S. "Depression is an inflammatory disease." Journal Watch

81

Psychiatry.2010 Mar.

Dowlati Y, Herrmann N, Swardfager W, Liu H, Sham L, Reim EK, Lanctôt KL. "A meta-analysis of cytokines in major depression." Biol Psychiatry. 2010 Mar 1;67(5):446-57; "This meta-analysis reports **significantly higher concentrations of the proinflammatory cytokines TNF-alpha and IL-6 in depressed subjects** compared with control subjects." [pentoxifylline reduces TNF-alpha and IL-6]

Akhondzadeh S, Fallah J, Mohammadi MR, Imani R, Mohammadi M, Salehi B, Ghanizadeh A, Raznahan M, Mohebbi-Rasa S, Rezazadeh SA, Forghani S. "Double-blind placebo-controlled trial of pentoxifylline added to risperidone: effects on aberrant behavior in children with autism." Prog Neuropsychopharmacol Biol Psychiatry. 2010 Feb 1;34(1):32-6.

Müller N, Schwarz MJ. "Antiinflammatory treatment approaches in major depression." European Psychiatry. 2010;25(sup1):120; "a statistically significant therapeutic effect of the COX-2 inhibitor on depressive symptoms in a randomized double blind pilot add-on study"; "Another randomized double-blind study in fifty depressed patients suffering from MD also showed an statistically significant better outcome of the COX-2 inhibitor celecoxib plus fluoxetine compared to fluoxetine alone."

Samsam M. "Role of inflammation in neurological and psychiatric disorders." Anti-Inflammatory & Anti-Allergy Agents in Medicinal Chemistry. 2010;9(3):166-169.

Masood A, Huang Y, Hajjhussein H, Xiao L, Li H, Wang W, Hamza A, Zhan CG, O'Donnell JM. "**Anxiolytic effects of phosphodiesterase-2 inhibitors** associated with increased cGMP signaling." J Pharmacol Exp Ther. 2009 Nov;331(2):690-9. [pentoxifylline primarily inhibits production of phosphodiesterase 4 – but somewhat inhibits production of phosphodiesterases 1,2, 3 & 5]

Pizzi C, Mancini S, Angeloni L, Fontana F, Manzoli L, Costa GM. "Effects of selective serotonin reuptake inhibitor therapy on endothelial function and inflammatory markers in patients with coronary heart disease." Clin Pharmacol Ther. 2009 Nov;86(5):527-32; "Levels of CRP and IL-6 ... decreased after 20 weeks of sertraline [a common antidepressant] treatment...."

Tobinick E. "Tumour necrosis factor modulation for treatment of Alzheimer's disease: rationale and current evidence." CNS Drugs. 2009 Sep 1;23(9):713-25; "... In the brain, among other functions, TNF [tumor necrosis factor] serves as a gliotransmitter, secreted by glial cells that envelope and surround synapses, which regulates synaptic communication between neurons. ... TNF may also play a role in endothelial and microvascular dysfunction in AD [Alzheimer's disease], and in amyloidogenesis and amyloid-induced memory dysfunction in AD. ... **Perispinal administration of etanercept, a potent anti-TNF fusion protein, produced sustained clinical improvement in a 6-month, open-label pilot study in patients with AD [Alzheimer's disease] ranging from mild to severe. Subsequent case studies have documented rapid clinical improvement following perispinal etanercept in both AD and primary progressive aphasia, providing evidence of rapidly reversible, TNF-dependent, pathophysiological mechanisms in AD and related disorders. ...**" [use of the less potent but safer pentoxifylline would require huge doses to be injected into the spinal canal]

Berthold-Losleben M, Heitmann S, Himmerich H. "Anti-inflammatory drugs in psychiatry." Inflamm Allergy Drug Targets. 2009 Sep;8(4):266-76; "cytokines such as tumor necrosis factor (TNF)-alpha, interferon (IFN)-alpha and IFN-gamma, contribute to the receptor resistance of neuropeptides, reduce the availability of amino acids which are needed for the synthesis of neurotransmitters or show neurotoxic effects"; "Cytokines are decisively involved in the pathophysiology of psychiatric disorders such as depression, schizophrenia or anorexia nervosa as well as in neurological disorders, respectively neurodegenerative diseases like Parkinson's or Alzheimer's."

Mösges R, Köberlein J, Heibges A, Erdtracht B, Klingel R, Lehmacher W; RHEO-ISHL Study Group. "Rheopheresis for **idiopathic sudden hearing** loss: results from a large prospective, multicenter, randomized, controlled clinical trial." Eur Arch Otorhinolaryngol. 2009 Jul;266(7):943-53; "**an effective treatment option**." [pentoxifylline is rheopheretic – blood-flow enhancing; sudden hearing loss usually is neurologic]

Himmerich H, Berthold-Losleben M, Pollmächer T. ["The relevance of the TNF-alpha system in psychiatric disorders"] [article in German; abstract in English is per www.pubmed.gov]. Fortschr Neurol Psychiatr. 2009 Jun;77(6):334-45; "TNF-alpha might contribute to the pathogenesis of these diseases by an activation of the hypothalamo-pituitary-adrenocortical (HPA) axis, an activation of neuronal serotonin transporters, the stimulation of the indoleamine 2,3-dioxygenase which leads to tryptophan depletion, by immunologically mediated destruction of neurons, or neurotoxic release of glutamate." [pentoxifylline reduces TNF-alpha]

Wei T, Sabsovich I, Guo TZ, Shi X, Zhao R, Li W, Geis C, Sommer C, Kingery WS, Clark DJ. "Pentoxifylline attenuates nociceptive sensitization and cytokine expression in a tibia fracture **rat** model of complex regional pain syndrome." Eur J Pain. **2009** Mar;13(3):253-62; "**pro-inflammatory cytokines contribute to the nociceptive and vascular sequelae of fracture and that PTX [pentoxifylline] treatment can reverse these** [Complex regional pain syndrome] **CRPS-like changes.**"

Uguz F, Akman C, Kucuksarac S, Tufekci O. "Anti-tumor necrosis factor-alpha therapy is associated with less frequent mood and anxiety disorders in patients with rheumatoid arthritis." Psychiatry Clin Neurosci. 2009 Feb;63(1):50-5; "83 consecutive patients with RA who were admitted to a rheumatology outpatient clinic."; "Mood and anxiety disorders were unrelated to sociodemographic features, disease-related factors, and medications for RA except anti-tumor necrosis factor-alpha (TNF-alpha). **These [mood and anxiety] disorders, however, were identified less frequently in patients with RA [rheumatoid arthritis] receiving anti-TNF-alpha drugs** compared to patients who did not receive such medications." [pentoxifylline reduces TNF-alpha]

Tobinick EL, Gross H. "Rapid improvement in verbal fluency and aphasia following perispinal etanercept in Alzheimer's disease." BMC Neurol. 2008 Jul 21;8:27; "**... Recent clinical studies point to rapid and sustained clinical, cognitive, and behavioral improvement in both Alzheimer's disease and primary progressive aphasia following weekly perispinal administration of etanercept, a TNF-alpha inhibitor** that acts by blocking the binding of this cytokine to its receptors. This outcome is concordant with recent basic science studies suggesting that TNF-alpha functions in vivo as a gliotransmitter that regulates synaptic function in the brain. ... In addition, **rapid improvement in verbal fluency and aphasia in two patients with dementia, beginning minutes after perispinal etanercept administration, is documented**. ..." [use of the less potent but safer pentoxifylline to reduce TNF-alpha would require huge doses to be injected – apparently weekly – into the spinal canal]

Bruce TO. "Comorbid depression in rheumatoid arthritis: pathophysiology and clinical implications." Curr Psychiatry Rep. 2008 Jun;10(3):258-64; "Inflammatory pathways may hold the key to a link between depression and RA [rheumatoid arthritis], and cytokines have been a major target of research in this area."

Tariq M, Ahmad M, Moutaery KA, Deeb SA. "Pentoxifylline ameliorates lithium-pilocarpine induced status epilepticus in young rats." Epilepsy Behav. 2008 Apr;12(3):354-65; "... Treatment with PTX [pentoxifylline] significantly ameliorated the frequency and severity of epileptic seizures in a dose-dependent manner. Our behavioral studies ... suggested **a significant reduction in anxiety, enhanced motor performance, and improved learning and memory in [pentoxifylline] PTX-treated rats**. ... The neuroprotective activity of PTX was accompanied by reduction in oxidative stress and reversal of SE [status epilepticus]-induced depletion of dopamine and 5-hydroxytryptamine in hippocampus and striatum. The results of **this study provide a good rationale to explore the prophylactic/ therapeutic potential of PTX [pentoxifylline] in SE [status epilepticus]**."

Salimi S, Fotouhi A, Ghoreishi A, Derakhshan MK, Khodaie-Ardakani MR, Mohammadi MR, Noorbala AA, Ahmadi-Abhari SA, Hajiazim M, Abbasi SH, Akhondzadeh S. "A placebo controlled study of the propentofylline added to risperidone in chronic schizophrenia." Prog Neuropsychopharmacol Biol Psychiatry. 2008 Apr 1;32(3):726-32; "... an 8-week double blind and placebo controlled trial. Eligible participants in this study were 50 patients with chronic schizophrenia. ... in the active phase of the illness .... Patients were allocated in a random fashion, 25 to risperidone 6 mg/day plus propentofylline 900 mg/day (300 mg TDS) and 25 to risperidone 6 mg/day plus placebo. ... **the combination of risperidone [a common antipsychotic] and propentofylline showed a significant superiority over risperidone alone in the treatment of positive [schizophrenic] symptoms, general psychopathology symptoms as well as PANSS [Positive and Negative Syndrome Scale] total scores**. The mean Extrapyramidal Symptoms Rating Scale [scores] for the placebo group were higher than in the propentofylline group over the trial. However, the differences were not significant. ..."

Dantzer R, O' Connor JC, Freund GG, Johnson RW, Kelley KW. "From inflammation to sickness and depression: when the immune system subjugates the brain." Nature Reviews Neuroscience. 2008;9:46-56.

Rook GAW, Lowry CA. "The hygiene hypothesis and psychiatric disorders." Trends in Immunology. 2008;29(4):150-158

Bhat AR, Wani MA, Kirmani A, Raina T, Alam S, Ramzan A. "Traumatic brain edema and survival – effective role of pentoxifylline." Biomed Res. 2008;19:9–12.
http://www.indmedica.com/journals.php?journalid=12&issueid=129&art icleid=1708&action=article ; "...case – control study of 108 **patients of traumatic brain edema** ... . The pentoxifylline was given as intravenous infusion of 300 mg (15 ml) dose in 300 ml normal saline over a period of 3 hours at a frequency of 8 hourly intervals. Alternatively 400 mg tablets at 8 hourly intervals were given through nasogastric tube. ... **mortality of 52.5% was observed in control-group of patients as compared to zero mortality in pentoxifylline-group. ... This study confirms the**

beneficial role of pentoxifylline in patients of traumatic brain edema by antagonizing a product of lipid peroxidation, malondialdehyde ...."

Hu R, Yuan BX, Su LZ, Wei XZ, Zhao LM, Kang J, Chen D. ["Pentoxifylline promotes learning and memory function of aging rats and mice with induced memory impairment"] [article in Chinese; abstract in English is per www.pubmed.gov]. Nan Fang Yi Ke Da Xue Xue Bao. 2007 Nov;27(11):1734-7.

Tyring S, Gottlieb A, Papp K, Gordon K, Leonardi C, Wang A, Lalla D, Woolley M, Jahreis A, Zitnik R, Cella D, Krishnan R. "Etanercept and clinical outcomes, fatigue, and depression in psoriasis: double-blind placebo-controlled randomised phase III trial." Lancet. 2006 Jan 7;367(9504):29-35; "Greater proportions of patients receiving etanercept [a TNF-alpha blocker] had at least a 50% improvement in Ham-D [Hamilton Depression Scale] or BDI [Beck Depression Inventory] at week 12 compared with the placebo group." [pentoxifylline reduces TNF-alpha]

Kanes SJ, Tokarczyk J, Siegel SJ, Bilker W, Abel T, Kelly MP. (2006). "Rolipram: A specific phosphodiesterase 4 inhibitor with potential antipsychotic activity." Neuroscience. 2006; 144 (1): 239–246. [pentoxifylline primarily inhibits production of phosphodiesterase 4]

American Psychiatric Association practice guidelines for the treatment of psychiatric disorders: Compendium 2006. Arlington, VA: American Psychiatric Publishing, 2006; pp.150, 168, 153 [re cerebral blood flow – which pentoxifylline enhances].

Lü LX, Guo SQ, Chen W, Li Q, Cheng J, Guo JH. ["Effect of clozapine and risperidone on serum cytokine levels in patients with first-episode paranoid schizophrenia"] [article in Chinese; abstract in English is per www.pubmed.gov]. Di Yi Jun Yi Da Xue Xue Bao. 2004 Nov;24(11):1251-4: "In patients treated with risperidone [a common antipsychotic], the levels of serum IL-6 ... after 4 weeks, TNF-alpha after 8 weeks ... were all significantly lowered ..."; "In clozapine [another antipsychotic] group, the levels of ... IL-6 ... after 6 months

were lowered significantly." [pentoxifylline inhibits production of IL-6 and TNF-alpha]

Maxwell CR, Kanes SJ, Abel T, Siegel SJ. "Phosphodiesterase inhibitors: a novel mechanism for receptor-independent antipsychotic medications." Neuroscience. 2004;129 (1): 101–7.

Boess FG, Hendrix M, van der Staay FJ, Erb C, Schreiber R, van Staveren W, de Vente J, Prickaerts J, Blokland A, Koenig G. "Inhibition of phosphodiesterase 2 increases neuronal cGMP, synaptic plasticity and memory performance." Neuropharmacology. 2004;47: 1081-1092. [pentoxifylline primarily inhibits production of phosphodiesterase 4 – but somewhat inhibits production of phosphodiesterases 1, 2, 3, & 5]

Urban B, Ustymowicz A, Bakunowicz-Lazarczyk A, Kretowska M. ["Effect of pentoxifylline on Doppler blood flow parameters in the central retinal artery and the short posterior ciliary arteries in adolescents with progressive myopia"] [short-sightedness] [article in Polish; abstract in English is per www.pubmed.gov] Klin Oczna. 2004;106(3):318-20.

Intriguingly, **a major US government meta-analysis published in 2004 found some support for the use of propentofylline in the treatment of vascular dementia ["some evidence of benefit for general cognitive function"; "Behavior/ mood outcomes ... were ... shown to be significantly different"] albeit not of pentoxifylline ["inconclusive"] – although the opening structured abstract of the report gave all the credit to the parent compound, pentoxifylline**. Santaguida P, Raina P, Booker L, Patterson C, Baldassarre F, Cowan D, Gauld M, Levine M, Unsal A. Pharmacological Treatment of Dementia: Evidence Reports/ Technology Assessments, No. 97. Rockville, MD: Agency for Healthcare Research and Quality (US); April 2004; the relevant data are in the "Results" chapter under the "Question 1" section then under the "Results of other agents" subsection.

Altschuler EL, Kast RE. "Bupropion in psoriasis and atopic dermatitis: decreased tumor necrosis factor-alpha?" Psychosom Med. 2003 Jul-Aug;65(4):719; "suggest that bupropion [a common antidepressant] works in these diseases by lowering the levels of the proinflammatory cytokine tumor necrosis factor-alpha (TNF). This would be consistent with our report that bupropion effected near complete clinical remission in patients with Crohn's disease ... and our finding that bupropion can lower TNF." [pentoxifylline reduces TNF-alpha]

Frampton M, Harvey RJ, Kirchner V. "Propentofylline for dementia." Cochrane Database Syst Rev. 2003;(2):CD002853. Review; "...There is limited evidence that **propentofylline might benefit cognition, global function and activities of daily living of people with Alzheimer's disease and/or vascular dementia... ."**

Sweitzer SM, Schubert P, DeLeo JA. "Propentofylline, a glial modulating agent, exhibits antiallodynic properties in a rat model of neuropathic pain." J Pharmacol Exp Ther. 2001 Jun;297(3):1210-7; "...**Systemic propentofylline was found to be equally effective in the attenuation of existing allodynia** [pain caused by a stimulus that usually does not cause pain] ... as in the prevention of allodynia in this rodent model of neuropathic pain. ... **Microglial and astrocytic activation was decreased by both peripheral and central administration of propentofylline in both preventative and existing allodynia paradigms. ..."** [according to Google Scholar, accessed on 11-FEB-11, this is the article on propentofylline most cited overall and per year]

Reichenberg A, Yirmiya R, Schuld A, Kraus T, Haack M, Morag A, Pollmächer T. "Arch Gen Psychiatry. 2001 May;58(5):445-52; "Significant positive correlations were found between cytokine secretion and endotoxin-induced anxiety ..., depressed mood ..., and decreases in memory performance ... ."

Treves TA, Korczyn AD. "Denbufylline in dementia: a double-blind controlled study." Dement Geriatr Cogn Disord. 1999 Nov-Dec;10(6):505-10; "... **patients who received denbufylline [a pentoxifylline analogue] tended to improve in terms of cognitive scores,** but the effects were not statistically significant. **MMSE [mini mental status examination] scores were found to be higher among**

89

patients who received denbufylline … ."

Kittner B. "Clinical trials of propentofylline in vascular dementia. European/ Canadian Propentofylline Study Group." Alzheimer Dis Assoc Disord. 1999 Oct-Dec;13 Suppl 3:S166-71; "…**Beneficial effects of propentofylline were consistently demonstrated in the domains of cognitive and global function for both VaD [vascular dementia] populations**; however, no treatment benefits could be demonstrated for activities of daily living … ."

Rao VS, Santos FA, Paula WG, Silva RM, Campos AR. "Effects of acute and repeated dose administration of caffeine and pentoxifylline on diazepam-induced mouse behavior in the hole-board test." Psychopharmacology (Berl). 1999 May;144(1):61-6; that **pentoxifylline exerts "anxiolytic-like activity similar to diazepam**."

Rother M, Erkinjuntti T, Roessner M, Kittner B, Marcusson J, Karlsson I. "Propentofylline in the treatment of Alzheimer's disease and vascular dementia: a review of phase III trials." Dement Geriatr Cogn Disord. 1998 Jul;9 Suppl 1:36-43. Review; "… 901 patients with mild-to-moderate AD and 359 patients with mild-to-moderate VaD were enrolled in four double-blind, placebo-controlled, randomized studies ranging in duration from 6 months to 56 weeks. **Propentofylline was found to provide consistent improvements over placebo in efficacy assessments for both AD [Alzheimer's Disease] and VaD [vascular dementia] patients.** In addition, results from a drug withdrawal study suggested **that propentofylline does not merely relieve dementia symptoms but slows the progression of the disease itself**. Propentofylline had a good safety profile and was generally well tolerated."

Mielke R, Ghaemi M, Kessler J, Kittner B, Szelies B, Herholz K, Heiss WD. "**Propentofylline** enhances cerebral metabolic response to auditory memory stimulation in Alzheimer's disease." J Neurol Sci. 1998 Jan 21;154(1):76-82; "…Twenty-eight subjects completed the 3-month study. The drug was well tolerated. In the active treatment group, **a significant increase of cerebral metabolic response to the memory task was** observed ... ."

Mielke R, Möller HJ, Erkinjuntti T, Rosenkranz B, Rother M, Kittner B. "Propentofylline in the treatment of vascular dementia and Alzheimer-type dementia: overview of phase I and phase II clinical trials." Alzheimer Dis Assoc Disord. 1998;12 Suppl 2:S29-35. Review; "...**PPF [propentofylline] yields clinically measurable improvements in the symptoms of dementia and prevents loss of stimulation-related increases in glucose metabolism over a treatment period of 3 months.** ..."

Bobon D, Breulet M, Gerard-Vandenhove MA, Guiot-Goffioul F, Plomteux G, Sastre-y-Hernandez M, Schratzer M, Troisfontaines B, von Frenckell R, Wachtel H. (1988). "Is phosphodiesterase inhibition a new mechanism of antidepressant action? A double blind double-dummy study between rolipram [a selective PDE-4] and desipramine [a common antidepressant] in hospitalized major and/or endogenous depressives." Eur Arch Psychiatry Neurol Sci. 1988;238 (1): 2–6.

Nickisch A, Heinemann M, Gross M. ["Drug therapy in sensorineural hearing loss in childhood"] [article in German; abstract in English is per www.pubmed.gov]. Laryngol Rhinol Otol (Stuttg). 1987 Dec;66(12):664-6.

Herskovits E, Vazquez A, Famulari A, Smud R, Tamaroff L, Fraiman H, Gonzalez AM, Vila J, Matera V. "Randomised trial of pentoxifylline versus acetylsalicylic acid plus dipyridamole in preventing transient ischaemic attacks." Lancet. 1981 May 2;1(8227):966-8; "... **The incidence of recurrent TIAs during 1 year of [multicenter] follow-up** was 28% in group A [36 patients receiving acetylsalicylic acid 1,050 mg/d & dipyridamole 150 mg/d] and **10% [ie, less than half as much] in group B [30 patients receiving pentoxifylline 1,200 mg/d]**; this difference was significant (p less than 0.05). The incidence of permanent strokes was similar in the two groups but distinctly lower (4.5%) than that usually reported after untreated TIA." [Follow-up: Herskovits E, Famulari A, Tamaroff L, Gonzalez AM, Vzquez A, Dominguez R, Fraiman H, Vila J,

Benjamin V, Matera V. "Comparative study of pentoxifylline vs antiaggregants in patients with transient ischaemic attacks." Acta Neurol Scand Suppl. 1989;127:31-5; "… Out of 235 **patients with recent cerebral transient ischaemic attacks**, 208 subjects were available for final evaluation after 6 months' randomised treatment with either pentoxifylline (PTX 1,200 mg/day) [100 patients] or a combination (ASAD) of acetylsalicylic acid (ASA, 1,050 mg/day) and dipyridamole (D, 150 mg/day) [108 patients]. … The **total rate of recurrence [of transient ischemic attacks] was 14% with PTX [pentoxifylline] as compared to 24.1% with ASAD {acetylsalicylic acid plus dipyridamole} treatment.**"]

Adisamito NA. "The clinical effect of pentoxifylline ('Trental') in the treatment of geriatric patients." Singapore Med J. 1979 Sep;20(3) Suppl 1:20-25.

Harwart D. "The treatment of chronic cerebrovascular insufficiency. A double-blind study with pentoxifylline ('Trental' 400)." Curr Med Res Opin. 1979;6(2):73-84.

CANCER (ONCOLOGIC) & BLOOD (HEMATOLOGIC) DISORDERS

The roles of pentoxifylline in oncology for the most part are not here discussed. The abstracts listed below outline that pentoxifylline apparently is directly apoptotic {encouraging "natural cell death"} for some cancers, helps otherwise healthy cells recover from therapeutic radiation, reduces successful metastasis {spread of cancer cells}, and, perhaps more importantly, sensitizes a variety of aberrant cells to the relatively immediate killing powers of radiation therapy as well as of chemotherapy agents.

Goel PN, Gude RP. "Delineating the anti-metastatic potential of pentoxifylline in combination with liposomal doxorubicin against breast cancer cells." Biomed Pharmacother. 2014 Mar;68(2):191-200; "…**The** combination regime [pentoxifylline & liposomal doxorubicin (Lipodox), an anthracycline anti-cancer agent] exhibited synergistic activity and inhibited cellular proliferation [in vitro & in vivo] to a greater extent with regard to each drug used alone."

Jacobs VL, De Leo JA. "Increased glutamate uptake in astrocytes via propentofylline results in increased tumor cell apoptosis using the CNS-1 glioma model." J Neurooncol. 2013 Aug;114(1):33-42; "…Primary **rodent** astrocytes and CNS-1 [rodent glioma] cells were co-cultured … in the presence of 5 mM glutamate. Cells were treated with propentofylline, an atypical synthetic methylxanthine known to increase glutamate transporter expression in astrocytes. …These data suggest that **astrocytes in the tumor microenvironment can be targeted by the drug, propentofylline, [negatively] affecting tumor cell growth.**"

Goel PN, Gude RP. "Curbing the focal adhesion kinase and its associated signalling events by pentoxifylline in MDA-MB-231 human breast cancer cells." Eur J Pharmacol. 2013 Aug 15;714(1-3):432-41; "... **[pentoxifylline] PTX exhibited anti-metastatic activity by affecting key processes such as proliferation, adhesion, migration, invasion and apoptosis.** ... PTX at sub-toxic doses lowers the level of activated FAK [Focal Adhesion Kinase], Extracellular Regulated Kinase or Mitogen Activated Protein Kinase (ERK/MAPK), Protein Kinase B (PKB/Akt) affecting cellular proliferation and survival. It blocks G1/S phase of cell cycle by inhibiting the expression of CyclinD1/Cdk6. Further, it modulates the activities of Rho GTP[guanosine triphosphate]ases and alters actin organisation resulting in decreased motility. **PTX [pentoxifylline] also delays tumor growth and inhibited blood vessel formation in vivo.** In purview of these findings, **PTX [pentoxifylline] surely qualifies as a suitable prospect in the intervention of breast cancer.**"

Kamran MZ, Gude RP. "Pentoxifylline inhibits melanoma tumor growth and angiogenesis by targeting STAT3 signaling pathway." Biomed Pharmacother. 2013 Jun;67(5):399-405; "... **Pentoxifylline (PTX), a phosphodiesterase inhibitor, has been shown to have anti-metastatic** or anti-angiogenic activity against many human cancers. ... we report that, PTX at sub-toxic doses can inhibit melanoma tumor growth and angiogenesis by targeting the STAT3 signaling pathway. ... PTX treatment significantly inhibited tumor growth and angiogenesis in intra-dermal xenograft **mouse** model in vivo without having any visible toxicity. ..."

Akudugu JM, Serafin AM, Böhm LJ. "In vitro radiosensitisation by pentoxifylline does not depend on p53 status." Int J Radiat Biol. 2013 Jun;89(6):462-70; "...Six human glioblastoma cell lines were tested for the effect of pentoxifylline treatment .... These results are at variance with view that pentoxifylline preferentially sensitises p53 mutant cells, and that sensitisation occurs only when cells are irradiated in the presence of the drug. The data suggest that **the effectiveness of pentoxifylline as radiosensitiser depends on the proportion of cells that are arrested in the G2/M [growth/ mitotic] phase transition following exposure to ionising radiation. ...**"

Fugler LA, Eades SC, Moore RM, Koch CE, Keowen ML. "Plasma matrix metalloproteinase activity in horses after intravenous infusion of lipopolysaccharide and treatment with matrix metalloproteinase inhibitors." Am J Vet Res. 2013 Mar;74(3):473-80; "... **Pentoxifylline** and oxytetracycline **appeared to be the most effective [matrix metalloproteinase] MMP-2 and MMP-9 inhibitor**s **[agents that encourage natural cell death]**, whereas doxycycline and flunixin meglumine were more effective at inhibiting MMP-2 activity than MMP-9 activity. ..."

Bravo-Cuellar A, Hernández-Flores G, Lerma-Díaz JM, Domínguez-Rodríguez JR, Jave-Suárez LF, De Célis-Carrillo R, Aguilar-Lemarroy A, Gómez-Lomeli P, Ortiz-Lazareno PC. "Pentoxifylline and the proteasome inhibitor MG132 induce apoptosis in human leukemia U937 cells through a decrease in the expression of Bcl-2 and Bcl-XL and phosphorylation of p65." J Biomed Sci. 2013 Feb 28;20(1):13; "...we investigated, in U937 human leukemia cells, the effects of **Pentoxifylline (PTX) and the MG132 proteasome inhibitor**, drugs that can disrupt the NF-kappaB

94

pathway. ... The two drugs used induce apoptosis per se, this **cytotoxicity was greater with combination of both drugs**. ... **this combination of drugs promotes the upregulation of the proapoptotic [natural cell death] genes and downregulation of antiapoptotic genes**. ..."

Ojeda PG, Perez AA, Ojeda L, Vargas-Uribe M, Rivas CI, Salas M, Vera JC, Reyes AM. "Non-competitive blocking of human GLUT1hexose transporter by methylxanthines reveals an exofacial regulatory binding site." Am J Physiol Cell Physiol. 2012 Sep;303(5):C530-9; "... The GLUT1 transporter has become an attractive target to **block glucose uptake in malignant cells** .... These results indicate that the **methylxanthines** do not bind to either the exofacial or endofacial D-glucose binding sites, but instead, they **interact at a different site accessible by the external face of the transporter**. Additionally, ... **only pentoxifylline** [but not caffeine or theophylline] **disturbed D-glucose for binding to the exofacial substrate site**. ...

Barancik M, Bohacova V, Gibalova L, Sedlak J, Sulova Z, Breier A. "Potentiation of anticancer drugs: effects of pentoxifylline on neoplastic cells." Int J Mol Sci. 2012;13(1):369-82; "... we investigated ... multidrug resistance (MDR) in mouse leukemia L1210/VCR cells. ... we conclude **that PTX [pentoxifylline] induces the sensitization of multidrug-resistant cells to VCR [vincristine, a common anticancer agent] via downregulation of P-gp [P-glycoprotein], stimulation of apoptosis [naural cell death] and reduction of MMPs [matrix metalloproteinases] released from drug-resistant L1210/VCR cells.** These facts bring new insights into the mechanisms of PTX [pentoxifylline] action on cancer cells."

Goel PN, Gude RP. "Unravelling the antimetastatic potential of pentoxifylline, a methylxanthine derivative in human MDA-MB-231 breast cancer cells." Mol Cell Biochem. 2011 Dec;358(1-2):141-51; "Pentoxifylline (PTX), a methylxanthine derivative is a non-steroidal immunomodulating agent with unique hemorheologic properties. ... PTX induced a G0-G1 cell-cycle arrest leading to apoptosis. Further, it affected adhesion to both the matrigel and collagen type-IV in a time- and dose-dependent manner. The PTX impeded the migration of MDA-MB-231 [M.D.Anderson-(highly) Metastatic Breast] cells and also **decreased the activities of both [matrix metalloproteinase] MMP-2 and MMP-9 [agents that encourage natural cell death]**. Thus, **PTX [pentoxifylline] at non-toxic doses affected cellular proliferation, adhesion, migration and invasion**. These results demonstrate its **anti-metastatic** effect on MDA-MB-231 cells ….

Woziwodzka A, Gwizdek-Wiśniewska A, Piosik J. "Caffeine, pentoxifylline and theophylline form stacking complexes with IQ-type heterocyclic aromatic amines." Bioorg Chem. 2011 Feb;39(1):10-7; "…demonstrated **a statistically significant reduction in HCAs [heterocyclic aromatic amines] mutagenic activity** in the presence of MTX [methylxanthines]." [pentoxifylline is a methylxanthine]

Gahlot S, Khan MA, Rishi L, Majumdar S. "Pentoxifylline augments TRAIL/Apo2L mediated apoptosis [natural programmed cell death] in cutaneous T cell lymphoma (HuT-78 and MyLa) by modulating the expression of antiapoptotic proteins and death receptors." Biochem Pharmacol. 2010 Dec 1;80(11):1650-61; "**PTX [pentoxifylline] can potentiate TRAIL-mediated apoptosis [natural cell death] through down-regulation of cell survival gene products and up-regulation of death receptors.**"

Asadpour M, Rasouly M, Ziaee M, Andalib S, Abadpour A, Doustar Y, Garjani A. "The effect of pentoxifylline on leukocyte accumulation and **angiogenesis** in air pouch model in rats." WorldPharma 2010. 16th World Congress of Basic and Clinical Pharmacology – Copenhagen - 17–23 July 2010; Abstract Book Supplement; pp.4-5; www.worldpharma2010.org/onsite_abstracts.pdf; "… Inflammation was produced by injection of carrageenan … Meanwhile pentoxifylline exerts antiangiogenesis effect with 10 mg/kg, 43% ($P<0.001$) and 40 mg/kg 15% ($P<0.05$) significantly but with 20 mg/kg induced angiogenesis 6% with no significance. …" [the question of **whether pentoxifylline is or is not antiangiogenic or may be synergistic with other antiangiogenesis agents** (eg, thalidomide) has been debated since about 2000; this article raises the possibility that a low dose and a high dose pentoxifylline might be very different than a moderate dose]

Bravo-Cuellar A, Ortiz-Lazareno PC, Lerma-Diaz JM, Dominguez-Rodriguez JR, Jave-Suarez LF, Aguilar-Lemarroy A, del Toro-Arreola S, de Celis-Carrillo R, Sahagun-Flores JE, de Alba-Garcia JE, Hernandez-Flores G. "Sensitization of cervix cancer cells to Adriamycin by Pentoxifylline induces an increase in apoptosis and a decrease in senescence." Mol Cancer. 2010 May 19;9:114; **"PTX [pentoxifylline] is a good inducer of apoptosis [natural cell death]** but does not induce senescence [aging]."

Fan S, Smith ML, Rivet DJ 2nd, Duba D, Zhan Q, Kohn KW, Fornace AJ Jr, O'Connor PM. "Disruption of p53 function sensitizes breast cancer MCF-7 cells to cisplatin and pentoxifylline." Cancer Res. 1995 Apr 15;55(8):1649-54; "...**The G2 [2nd** phase of cellular growth just before mitosis] **checkpoint inhibitor pentoxifylline exhibited synergism with CDDP** [cisplatin, a chemotherapy agent] **in killing MCF-7/E6 cells [a** breast cancer cell line] **but did not affect sensitivity of the control cells. ... a combination of CDDP and pentoxifylline is capable of synergistic and preferential killing of p53-defective tumor cells that do not readily undergo apoptosis** [natural programmed cell death]." [according to Google Scholar, accessed on 11-FEB-11, this is the article on pentoxifylline, other than a 1987 review, 4th most cited overall and 2nd most cited per year]

INFECTIOUS (VIRAL, BACTERIAL, & FUNGAL) DISORDERS

The abstracts listed below note the observed anti-infection activities of pentoxifylline – most likely by a number of mechanisms, including helping to carry other agents toward the infection.

Jiménez-Luévano MA, Lerma-Díaz JM, Hernández-Flores G, Jiménez-Partida MA, Bravo-Cuellar A. "Addition of pentoxifylline to pegylated interferon-alpha-2a and ribavirin improves sustained virological response to chronic hepatitis C virus: a randomized clinical trial." Ann Hepatol. 2013 Mar;12(2):248-55; "…**pentoxifylline (PTX) possesses antiviral and hepatoprotector properties**. … Seventy two patients of both genders were studied in a randomized fashion … . During 48 weeks, control group patients were treated with PEG INFalpha- 2a plus ribavirin. PTX [pentoxifylline] was administered to Experimental Group patients prior to the treatment. … **SVR [sustained virological response] in the experimental group increased significantly** (p < 0.05) when compared with standard therapy alone. …"

Salgado D, Zabaleta TE, Hatch S, Vega MR, Rodriguez J. "Use of pentoxifylline in treatment of children with dengue hemorrhagic fever." Pediatr Infect Dis J. 2012 Jul;31(7):771-3; "… a pilot study evaluating **pentoxifylline**'s effect on 55 children with **dengue hemorrhagic fever**. … our findings support … **its potential use in severe infection**."

Tsirilakis K, Kim C, Vicencio AG, Andrade C, Casadevall A, Goldman DL. "Methylxanthine Inhibit Fungal Chitinases and Exhibit Antifungal Activity." Mycopathologia. 2012 Mar;173(2-3):83-91; "Chitinases are necessary for fungal cell wall remodeling and cell replication. … Fungi demonstrated variable chitinase activity and incubation with methylxanthines (0.5-10 mM) resulted in a dose-dependent decrease in this activity. All fungi tested, except for Candida spp., demonstrated growth inhibition in the presence of methylxanthines at a concentration of 10 mM. … **C. neoformans and Aspergillus fumigatus treated with pentoxifylline also exhibited abnormal cell morphology**. …Our results highlight **the potential utility of targeting chitinases in the development of novel antifungal therapies**."

Costantini TW, Deree J, Peterson CY, Putnam JG, Woon T, Loomis WH, Bansal V, Coimbra R. "Pentoxifylline modulates p47phox activation and **downregulates neutrophil oxidative burst** through PKA-dependent and -independent mechanisms." Immunopharmacol Immunotoxicol. 2010 Mar;32(1):82-91; "…Pentoxifylline (PTX) has been proven to be an inhibitor of fMLP-induced neutrophil (PMN) oxidative burst and is

thought to function by increasing cAMP and Protein kinase A (PKA). …
PTX [pentoxifylline] attenuates activation of signaling molecules
involved in activation of p47phox and suppresses the subsequent assembly
of the NADPH [nicotinamide adenine dinucleotide phosphate] machinery
through both PKA-dependent and PKA-independent mechanisms."

Krakauer T. "Therapeutic down-modulators of Staphylococcal
superantigen-induced inflammation and toxic shock." Toxins. 2010;
2:1963-1983; "Pentoxyfylline … interference with intracellular pathways
affects leukocyte adhesion and cytokine production. Pentoxyfylline
inhibited SEB-[Staphylococcal enterotoxin B]or TSST-1- [toxic shock
syndrome toxin 1] induced toxic shock, as well as cytokine and chemokine
release [15,95]. Dexamethasone, **pentoxyfylline**, doxycycline, and
rapamycin are FDA-approved drugs used for other indications, and have
been **in clinical use for many years with a proven safety record**"; "The
ability to **stop the cytokine cascade and the inflammatory events
initiated by cytokines early appears to be critical in preventing toxic
shock**. However, the tissue damage from cytokine storm lingers and
**resolution of inflammation, especially in the lungs, appears to be
critical in preventing shock**" [pentoxifylline allows then stops cytokine
crisis].

Kucherov II, Rytik PG, Podol'skaya IA, Mistryukova LO, Korjev MO.
"Novel inhibitors of HIV discovered among existing classes of
pharmaceutical compounds indicated for unrelated clinical indications."
Curr Pharm Des. 2009;15(11):1187-90: "and Trental **[pentoxifylline]
may become valid candidates for inclusion into antiviral regimens**."

Sebastian L, Desai A, Madhusudana SN, Ravi V. "Pentoxifylline inhibits
replication of Japanese encephalitis virus: a comparative study with
ribavirin." Int J Antimicrob Agents. 2009 Feb;33(2):168-73;
"**pentoxifylline possesses broad-spectrum antiviral activity against a
range of RNA and DNA viruses**. … The present study was designed to
investigate the antiviral activity of pentoxifylline against JEV in vitro and
in vivo."

Wanchu A, Bhatnagar A, Bambery P, Singh S, Varma S. "Prevention of opportunistic infections in HIV infection by pentoxiphylline." Indian J Med Res. 2006 Dec;124(6):705-8; "**Pentoxiphylline therapy in HIV infected individuals**, who were free of opportunistic infections, improved their body weight, **minimized opportunistic infections, increased and sustained CD4 counts**. Given the low cost of the drug it could be recommended for the use in individuals who are at a high risk of developing opportunistic infections."

Rao FV1, Andersen OA, Vora KA, Demartino JA, van Aalten DM. "Methylxanthine drugs are chitinase inhibitors: investigation of inhibition and binding modes." Chem Biol. 2005 Sep;12(9):973-80; "...**competitive inhibitors against a fungal family 18 chitinase, with pentoxifylline being the most potent ... .**"

Bermejo Martin JF, Jimenez JL, Muńoz-Fernández A. "Pentoxifylline and severe acute respiratory syndrome (SARS): a drug to be considered." Med Sci Monit. 2003 Jun;9(6):SR29-34; "**The antiinflammatory, antiviral, immunomodulatory and bronchodilatory effects of PTX [pentoxifylline] along with its low cost and toxicity, make it a promising drug to be considered for SARS [severe acute respiratory syndrome] treatment ... .**"

Staubach KH, Schröder J, Stüber F, Gehrke K, Traumann E, Zabel P. "Effect of pentoxifylline in severe sepsis: results of a randomized, double-blind, placebo-controlled study." Arch Surg. 1998 Jan;133(1):94-100; "... Fifty-one surgical **patients with severe sepsis** were randomized to receive pentoxifylline continuously (27 patients) or saline infusion as placebo (24 patients). ... Patients received pentoxifylline (1 mg/kg of body weight per hour; maximum, 1,800 mg/d) during 28 days or until they were discharged from the intensive care unit or died. ... **Hospital mortality was 41% (11/27) in the pentoxifylline group and 54% (13/24) in the placebo group**. The multiple organ dysfunction score decreased in patients receiving pentoxifylline 4 days after diagnosis of sepsis compared with placebo-treated patients; a significant difference was reached on day 14 ...
. The PaO2/FIO2 (fraction of inspired oxygen) ratio was significantly

improved in pentoxifylline-treated patients on days 14 and 17 ... and the pressure-adjusted heart rate was significantly improved on day 6 ... compared with the placebo group. ... **Continuous intravenous administration of pentoxifylline beneficially influenced cardiopulmonary dysfunction in patients with sepsis without adverse effects. ...**"

Hand WL, Hand DL. "Influence of pentoxifylline and its derivatives on antibiotic uptake and superoxide generation by human phagocytic cells." Antimicrob Agents Chemother. 1995 Jul;39(7):1574-9; "**The ability of pentoxifylline to augment the entry of antibiotics into neutrophils** has important therapeutic implications. The consequences of this phenomenon might include improved intracellular bactericidal activity as well as efficient antibiotic delivery and release at sites of infection."

Di Perri G, Di Perri IG, Monteiro GB, Bonora S, Hennig C, Cassatella M, Micciolo R, Vento S, Dusi S, Bassetti D, Concia E. "Pentoxifylline as a supportive agent in the treatment of cerebral malaria in children." J Infect Dis. 1995 May;171(5):1317-22.

Lauterbach R, Pawlik D, Tomaszczyk B, Cholewa B. "Pentoxifylline treatment of sepsis of premature infants: preliminary clinical observations." Eur J Pediatr. 1994 Sep;153(9):672-4.

Amvros'eva TV, Votiakov VI, Andreeva OT, Vladyko GV, Nikolaeva SN, Orlova SV, Azarova IA, Zgirovskaia AA. ["New properties of trental as an inhibitor of viral activity with a wide range of activity"] [article in Russian; abstract in English is per www.pubmed.gov]. Vopr Virusol. 1993 Sep-Dec;38(5):230-3; "investigations were done in cell cultures and laboratory animals using laboratory strains (including drug-resistant ones) of 13 viruses, causative agents of human and animal infections"; "It was highly active against 5 viruses: herpes simplex virus (including its acyclovir-resistant strain), vaccinia virus (including its methisazone-resistant strain), rotavirus and tick-borne encephalitis virus"; " trental **[pentoxifylline] was an effective broad spectrum virus inhibitor.**"

Schönharting MM, Schade UF. "The effect of pentoxifylline in septic shock – new pharmacologic aspects of an established drug." J Med. 1989;20(1):97-105; " … **pentoxifylline will also be of great benefit in different models of animal sepsis, including both gram positive and gram negative bacteria**. … survival rates are significantly increased in the pentoxifylline group when compared with the controls, which is paralleled by **a decrease in germ counts**. … this drug interferes with pathologic granulocyte-endothelium interactions …, both **downregulating intravasal granulocyte hyperreactivity** as well as **stimulating antiaggregatory activity of the vessel endothelium**. …"

FIBROTIC DISORDERS (INCLUDING PEYRONIE'S DISEASE)

The abstracts listed below focus more on radiation-induced fibrosis than on the fibrosis-related problems with penile erection [Peyronie's Disease].

Alizadeh M, Karimi F, Fallah MR. "Evaluation of verapamil efficacy in peyronie's disease comparing with pentoxifylline." Glob J Health Sci. 2014 Sep 18;6(7 Spec No):38292; "…The [90] patients were randomly divided into 3 groups. First group received pentoxifylline orally at a dose of 400 mg three times a day, in the second group verapamil (10 mg every other week for up to 12 sessions) was injected into the lesion and the third group received both treatments in combination. … **there was no significant difference between two groups using verapamil or pentoxifylline, but there was a significant improvement in combination therapy group**. …"

Wong RK, Bensadoun RJ, Boers-Doets CB, Bryce J, Chan A, Epstein JB, Eaby-Sandy B, Lacouture ME. "Clinical practice guidelines for the prevention and treatment of acute and late radiation reactions from the MASCC Skin Toxicity Study Group." Support Care Cancer. 2013 Oct;21(10):2933-48; "…**For patients with established radiation-induced telangiectasia and fibrosis, the panel suggests the use of … pentoxifylline and vitamin E for the reduction of fibrosis**."

Jacobson G, Bhatia S, Smith BJ, Button AM, Bodeker K, Buatti J. "Randomized trial of pentoxifylline and vitamin E vs standard follow-up after breast irradiation to prevent breast fibrosis, evaluated by tissue compliance meter." Int J Radiat Oncol Biol Phys. 2013 Mar 1;85(3):604-8; "...This study of **postirradiation breast cancer patients treated with PTX [pentoxifylline** 400 mg 3 times daily]/ vitamin E [400 IU daily] [for 6 months] or standard follow-up indicated **a significant difference in radiation-induced fibrosis** as measured by TCM [tissue compliance meter at 18 months]. ... The treatment was safe and well tolerated. ..."

Hamama S, Gilbert-Sirieix M, Vozenin MC, Delanian S. "Radiation-induced enteropathy: Molecular basis of pentoxifylline-vitamin E anti-fibrotic effect involved TGF-$\beta(1)$ cascade inhibition." Radiother Oncol. 2012 Dec;105(3):305-12.; "... primary smooth muscle cells isolated from intestinal samples isolated from humans with radiation enteropathy were incubated with pentoxifylline, trolox (vit. E hydrophilic analogous) or their combination. ... In vitro, **pentoxifylline and trolox [vitamin E] synergize to inhibit TGF [Transforming growth factor]-β1 protein and mRNA [messenger ribonucleic acid] expression. This inhibitory action is mediated at the transcriptional level** ....

Türke B, Balázs C. ["Treatment of pretibial myxoedema with pentoxifylline"]. [article in Hungarian; abstract in English is per www.pubmed.gov] Orv Hetil. 2012 Oct 28;153(43):1719-22; "... the case of a 34-year-old male patient with pretibial myxoedema treated successfully with pentoxifylline. ... He received first intradermal, then intravenous and, finally, oral pentoxifylline, which resulted in a regression of the dermatological symptoms. The beneficial effect of pentoxifylline might be explained by its inhibitory effect on proinflammatory cytokines and proliferation of fibroblasts, and the production of glycosaminoglycan. ... **pentoxifylline can be an effective and safe treatment of pretibial myxoedema.**"

Smith JF, Shindel AW, Huang Y-C, Clavijo RI, Flechner L, Breyer BN, Eisenberg ML, Lue TF. "Pentoxifylline treatment and penile calcifications in men with Peyronie's disease." Asian J Andrology. Mar 2011;13:322-325; "...71 men (mean age: 51.9 years) with Peyronie's Disease and sonographic evidence of calcification were identified. Of them, 62 of these men were treated with PTX [pentoxifylline] for a mean duration of 1 year, and nine with vitamin E or no treatment. Improvement or stabilization in calcium burden at follow-up was noted in 57 (91.9%) of men treated with PTX versus four (44.4%) of those not treated with PTX (P,0.001). PTX users were much less likely to have a subjective worsening of their clinical condition (25.0% versus 78.3%, P50.002). **Treatment with PTX [pentoxifylline] appeared to stabilize or reduce calcium content in Peyronie's Disease plaques. ...**"

Mehrotra R, Singh H, Gupta S, Singh M, Jain S. "Pentoxifylline therapy in the management of oral submucous fibrosis." Asian Pac J Cancer Prev. 2011;12(4):971-4; "...**Oral submucous fibrosis** is a common premalignant condition in the Indian subcontinent ... . 75 patients suffering from oral submucous fibrosis were randomly divided into two groups A and B. Group A patients received placebo, while Group B patients received 400 mg **Pentoxifylline** for a period of 7 months. ... The improvement in total ... score was 25% in group A and 49.15% in group B. ...**Treatment regimen of group B was more effective**. No significant side effects were seen. ..." [note that the dose used was one-third of the more common dose]

SKIN (DERMATOLOGIC) DISORDERS

The abstracts listed below note a wide array of skin disorders treated with pentoxifylline plus a more specific agent; apparently pentoxifylline helps in the delivery of both blood flow and perhaps another healing ingredient.

Rewale V, Prabhakar KR, Chitale AM."Pentoxifylline: a new armamentarium in diabetic foot ulcers." J Clin Diagn Res. 2014 Jan;8(1):84-6; "... Out of 67 patients 30 received pentoxyfylline and 32 were on traditional treatment and there was loss of follow-up in five cases.

… It was observed that **the patients on pentoxyfylline [400 mg tid] had early healing as compared to patients receiving only conventional treatment as evident on biopsy and Doppler. …"**

Hu L, Alexander C, Eastham A, Girouard S, Femia A, Vleugels RA. "Isolated facial vasculopathy responding to pentoxifylline." Poster #1051, 11 May 2013; International Investigative Dermatology meeting, Edinburgh, Scotland.

Jull AB, Arroll B, Parag V, Waters J. "Pentoxifylline for treating venous leg ulcers." Cochrane Database Syst Rev. 2012 Dec 12; "… **Pentoxifylline is an effective adjunct to compression bandaging for treating venous ulcers and may be effective in the absence of compression. …"**

Mun JH, Jwa SW, Song M, Kim HS, Ko HC, Kim BS, Kim MB. "Extensive **pigmented purpuric dermatosis** successfully treated with pentoxifylline." Ann Dermatol. 2012 Aug;24(3):363-5. http://www.ncbi.nlm.nih.gov/pmc/articles/PMC3412251/?tool=pubmed; "... pentoxifylline, … is supposed to affect T-cell adherence to endothelial cells and keratinocytes … . The therapeutic effect of pentoxifylline [400 mg twice a day] was obvious in these two patients because the lesions in both disappeared within 1 and 2 months of treatment. During follow-up (5 months for case 1 and 2 years for case 2), recurrence was not observed. …" [note that the dose used was two-thirds of the more common dose]

Uzoma MA, Wilkerson MG, Carr VL, Westhoven GS, Raimer SA. "Pentoxifylline and cyclosporine in the treatment of febrile ulceronecrotic Mucha-Habermann disease." Pediatr Dermatol. 2014 Jul-Aug;31(4):525-7; "… we are presenting the first case of FUMHD [**febrile ulceronecrotic Mucha-Habermann disease] treated with pentoxifylline** [which] … may be of therapeutic benefit … in part by suppressing tumor necrosis factor-alpha … .

el-Darouti M, Marzouk S, Abdel Hay R, el-Tawdy A, Fawzy M, Leheta T, Gammaz H, Al Gendy N. "The use of sulfasalazine and pentoxifylline (low-cost anti-tumour necrosis factor drugs) as adjuvant therapy for the treatment of pemphigus vulgaris: a comparative study." Br J Dermatol. 2009 Aug;161(2):313-9; **"The use of PTX [pentoxifylline] and SSZ [sulfasalazine] as adjuvant therapy in the treatment of PV [pemphigus vulgaris] induced a faster and more significant decrease in the serum level of TNF-alpha, and this decrease was associated with rapid clinical improvement."**

Chartier M, Falanga V. "Healing of ulcers due to cryofibrinogenemia with colchicine and high-dose pentoxifylline." Am J Clin Dermatol. 2009;10(1):39-42; "The patient continued to have ulcerations despite efforts to control his high blood pressure, cold avoidance, local wound care, and treatment with pentoxifylline 800 mg three times daily. However, when colchicine 0.6 mg twice daily was added to the patient's care, this led to rapid healing of his ulcerations. He has remained ulcer free for 2 years taking the combination of colchicine and high-dose pentoxifylline. Efforts to reduce the dose of these agents have repeatedly led to recurrences, and remission has promptly followed re-establishment of the combination. To our knowledge, this is the first report documenting use of **the combination of colchicine and high-dose pentoxifylline to successfully treat ulcers due to cryofibrinogenemia.**"

Torres-Alvarez B, Castanedo-Cazares JP, Moncada B. "Pentoxifylline in the treatment of actinic prurigo. A preliminary report of 10 patients." Dermatology 2004;208:198-201; "Actinic prurigo (AP) is a chronic familial photodermatosis … . **Relief in pruritus was evident after 1 month of treatment and was maintained while receiving PTX [pentoxifylline]. …** PTX was useful **in the treatment of our actinic prurigo patients. It may induce a complete or partial remission of lesions and allow a decrease in the use of topical corticosteroids."** [the article that began this line of small case series was: Rubel DM, Wood G, Rosen R, Jopp-McKay A. "Generalised granuloma annulare successfully treated with pentoxifylline." Australas J Dermatol. 1993;34(3):103-8; **"…a patient with a ten year history of generalised GA [granuloma annulare], who showed dramatic clearing of the majority of papules after four weeks of treatment with pentoxifylline.** This drug has shown

106

promising results in the treatment of many dermatologic disorders including necrobiosis lipoidica diabeticorum, leukocytoclastic vasculitis and Raynaud's phenomenon. Pentoxifylline ... offers a well-tolerated and effective alternative ... ."; see also: Rubio FA, Robayna G, Pizarro A, de Lucas R, Herranz P, Casado M. "Actinic granuloma and vitiligo treated with pentoxifylline."Int J Dermatol. 1998 Dec;37(12):958-60.

Wahba-Yahav AV. "Intractable chronic furunculosis: prevention of recurrences with pentoxifylline." Acta Derm Venereol. 1992 Nov;72(6):461-2; "... A 60-year-old ... suffered from chronic recurrent furunculosis since the age of 30. In recent years, his condition had become increasingly severe and the recurrences increasingly frequent. Different measures including continuous therapy with large doses of systemic antibiotics for a period of 6 months failed to prevent the recurrences. Oral treatment with pentoxifylline 400 mg t.i.d. was prescribed, and 2 months later the patient experienced a dramatic and complete remission of his furunculosis. Six months later he was still totally free of lesions while continuing to take the same medication. **Pentoxifylline may provide a new and effective approach ... management of patients with chronic recurrent furunculosis.**"

RADIATION-INDUCED & TOXIN-INDUCED DISORDERS

The abstracts listed below note that pentoxifylline helps in the delivery of both blood flow and perhaps another healing ingredient – frequently an analogue of vitamin E – to tissues damaged by radiation.

Kahenasa N, Sung EC, Nabili V, Kelly J, Garrett N, Nishimura I. "Resolution of pain and complete healing of mandibular osteoradionecrosis using pentoxifylline and tocopherol: a case report." Oral Surg Oral Med Oral Pathol Oral Radiol. 2012 Apr;113(4):e18-23; "... Osteoradionecrosis (ORN) is a late effect of RIF [radiation-induced fibroatrophy] ... that can occur in 20% of patients irradiated for head and neck cancer. … we present a case of … **ORN [osteoradionecrosis] of the left posterior lingual mandibular cortex that was successfully treated and resolved with 6 months of pentoxifylline 400 mg twice a day and tocopherol 1,000 IU every day**." [note that the dose used was two-thirds of the more common dose]

Weintraub JA, Bennett J, Gaspar LE. Successful treatment of **radiation-induced optic neuropathy**." Pract Radiat Oncol. Jan 2011;1(1):40-44; "…pentoxifylline has been shown to down-regulate the expression of important cytokines that lead to radiation injury, such as transforming growth factor-β1. … **Although it is difficult to determine which treatment had the greatest effect, this combination of steroids, pentoxifylline, vitamin E, and anticoagulants had a beneficial effect in our patient [despite a 2-week delay in treatment, when sparse past literature has suggested a 72-hour window for initiation of treatment in this emergent condition]**."

Aziz TA. "Concentration-dependant antioxidant activity of pentoxifylline in nitrite-induced hemoglobin oxidation model." Iraqi J Pharm Sci. 2011;20(1):66-69; "**Free radical formation in heme proteins is recognized as a factor in mediating the toxicity of many chemicals. … pentoxifylline can effectively, in concentration dependent pattern, attenuate sodium nitrite-induced Hb [hemoglobin] oxidation in vitro**."

Kulkarni S. "Combination treatment of gamma-tocotrienol with pentoxifylline improves radioprotective efficacy of GT3 in mouse model." Chemical and Biological Defense Science and Technology Conference, 2010 Nov 15; poster presentation T25-006; compare: Berbée M, Fu Q, Garg S, Kulkarni S, Kumar KS, Hauer-Jensen M. "Pentoxifylline enhances the radioprotective properties of γ-tocotrienol: Differential effects on the hematopoietic, gastrointestinal and vascular systems." Radiat Res. 2011 Mar;175(3):297-306; "… The vitamin E analog γ-tocotrienol (GT3) is a potent radioprotector and mitigator. … **Mice** were injected subcutaneously with vehicle, GT3 [400 mg/kg 24 h before total-body irradiation (TBI)], PTX [pentoxifylline] (200 mg/kg 30 min before TBI), or GT3+PTX before being exposed to 8.5-13 Gy ["Gray unit" =

absorbed radiation dose of ionizing radiation] TBI [total body irradiation]. … **Combined treatment with GT3 [a vitamin E analogue] and PTX [pentoxifylline] increased postirradiation survival over that with GT3 alone**. …"

Ranjbar A, Sharifzadeh M, Golestani A, Ghazi-Khansari M, Baeeri M, Abdollahi M. "Protection by pentoxifylline of malathion-induced toxic stress and mitochondrial damage in rat brain." Hum Exp Toxicol 2010 Oct; 29(10):851-864; "oxidative damage is at least in part the mechanism of **toxicity of malathion in the mitochondria that can be recovered by PTX [pentoxifylline]** comparable to AT [alpha-tocopherol]."

Goans RE, Hourigan PE. "Medical treatment of radiological casualties." Partial-body radiation diagnostic biomarkers and medical management of radiation injury workshop - 2008 May 05; "**During the third and fourth week [after radiologic exposure] when small vessel occlusion and fibrosis will be occurring, Pentoxifylline has been used successfully in the US to increase blood flow**"; manuscript at www.afrri.usuhs.mil/pb_rad_workshop/pdf/goans_abs2.pdf ; conference synopsis at Radiat Res. 2010 Feb;173(2):245-53.

Brown, SL. "Pharmacological agents that reduce radiation injury to normal tissue and do not reduce anti-tumor effect of radiation." Advanced Radiation Therapeutics - Radiation Injury Mitigation Workshop; sponsored by the [US] National Cancer Institute. 2010 Jan 25; lists pentoxifylline under "Other Promising Approaches."

Delanian S, Lefaix JL, Maisonobe T, Salachas F, Pradat PF. "Significant clinical improvement in radiation-induced lumbosacral polyradiculopathy by a treatment combining pentoxifylline, tocopherol, and clodronate (Pentoclo)." J Neurol Sci. 2008 Dec 15;275(1-2):164-6; Two patients with progressive worsening RI [radiation induced] lumbosacral polyradiculopathy experienced over several years a **significant clinical improvement in their neurological sensorimotor symptoms with long-term pentoxifylline- tocopherol- clodronate treatment**, and good safety.

Jarrett DG, Sedlak RG, Dickerson WE, Reeves GI. "Medical treatment of radiation injuries: Current US status." Radiation Measurements. 2007 JUL-AUG;42(6-7):1063-1074; excerpts ?from this edition or from a previous edition? at http://www.afrri.usuhs.mil/outreach/summary.htm ; "Truncal Lesions. ... **Lesions caused by highly penetrating radiations should be treated with drugs intended to improve microcirculation (pentoxifylline-trental) whenever adequate perfusion at affected and surrounding tissues exists.**"

SEXUAL (REPRODUCTIVE) DISORDERS, RELATIVE OMISSION OF DATA HERE

The abstract listed below only touches upon the vast literature on the roles of pentoxifylline in reproductive medicine. Almost from the beginning pentoxifylline has been investigated for and used in the amelioration of male and female breeding problems – but most of the literature has been in veterinary rather than in (human) medical journals.

Aleyasin A, Aghahosseini M, Mohseni M, Mahdavi A. "Effects of pentoxifylline and vitamin E on pregnancy rate in infertile women treated by ZIFT [zygote intra fallopian transfer]: a randomized clinical trial." Iranian J of Reprod Med. 2009 Autumn;7(4):175-179; "**the rate of pregnancy was significantly higher in PTX [pentoxifylline] and vit. E group** (57.14% vs 39.29%, p=0.01)...."

A FINAL WORD

The following article, from some veterinarians' point of view, perhaps says it all:

Marks SL, Merchant S, Foil C. "**Pentoxifylline: wonder drug?**" J Am Anim Hosp Assoc. 2001 May-Jun;37(3):218-9.

\#